BOTTOM LINE'S GUIDE TO
BRAIN-BUILDING
SECRETS

Keep your brain HEALTHY and memory STRONG

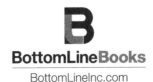

BottomLineBooks

BottomLineInc.com

ISBN 0-88723-793-2

Bottom Line Books® publishes the advice of expert authorities in many fields. These opinions may at times conflict as there are often different approaches to solving problems. The use of this material is no substitute for health, legal, accounting or other professional services. Consult competent professionals for answers to your specific questions.

Telephone numbers, addresses, prices, offers and websites listed in this book are accurate at the time of publication, but they are subject to frequent change.

Bottom Line Books® is a registered trademark of Bottom Line Inc., 3 Landmark Square, Suite 201, Stamford, CT 06901

BottomLineInc.com

Bottom Line Books® is an imprint of Bottom Line Inc., publisher of print periodicals, e-letters and books. We are dedicated to bringing you the best information from the most knowledgeable sources in the world. Our goal is to help you gain greater wealth, better health, more wisdom, extra time and increased happiness.

Printed in the United States of America

Contents

4. HELP FOR CANCER AND OTHER BRAIN DANGERS

5. STROKE STOPPERS

6. BRAIN FITNESS

7. BRAIN FOODS AND SUPPLEMENTS

8. MEMORY BOOSTERS

9. SLEEP WELL FOR A HEALTHY BRAIN

10. HOW YOUR BRAIN CAN HEAL YOUR BODY

CHAPTER 1

Alzheimer's and Dementia Prevention and Risks

Dr. Kosik's Alzheimer's Prevention Plan: Six Powerful Secrets

Kenneth S. Kosik, MD, the Harriman Professor of Neuroscience Research and codirector of the Neuroscience Research Institute at the University of California, Santa Barbara, where he specializes in the causes and treatments of neurodegeneration, particularly Alzheimer's disease. Dr. Kosik is coauthor of *Outsmarting Alzheimer's*.

If someone told you that there was a pill with no side effects and strong evidence showing that it helps prevent Alzheimer's disease, would you take it? Of course, you would!

The truth is, there's no such "magic bullet," but most adults do have the ability to dramatically decrease their risk for this dreaded disease.

A window of opportunity: According to the latest scientific evidence, slowing or blocking Alzheimer's plaques (buildups of dangerous protein fragments), which are now known to develop years before memory loss and other symptoms are noticeable, could be the key to stopping this disease.

After researching Alzheimer's for more than 25 years, here are the habits that I incorporate into my daily routine to help prevent Alzheimer's...

STEP 1: **Make exercise exciting.** You may know that frequent exercise—particularly aerobic exercise, which promotes blood flow to the brain—is the most effective Alzheimer's prevention strategy. Unfortunately, many people become bored and stop exercising.

Scientific evidence: Because exercise raises levels of brain-derived neuro-trophic factor, it promotes the growth of new brain cells and may help prevent shrinkage of the hippocampus (a part of the brain involved in memory).

What I do: Most days, I spend 35 minutes on an elliptical trainer, followed by some weight training (increasing muscle mass helps prevent diabetes—an Alzheimer's risk factor). To break up the monotony, I go mountain biking on sunny days. I advise patients who have trouble sticking to an exercise regimen to try out the new virtual-reality equipment available in many gyms. While riding a stationary bike, for example, you can watch a monitor that puts you in the Tour de France!

Also helpful: To keep your exercise regimen exciting, go dancing. A recent 20-year study found that dancing reduced dementia risk more than any other type of exercise—perhaps because many types of dancing (such as tango, salsa and Zumba) involve learning new steps and aerobic activity. Do the type of dancing that appeals to you most.

STEP 2: **Keep your eating plan simple.** A nutritious diet is important for Alzheimer's prevention, but many people assume that they'll have to make massive changes, so they get overwhelmed and don't even try. To avoid this trap, keep it simple—all healthful diets have a few common elements, including an emphasis on antioxidant-rich foods (such as fruit and vegetables)…not too much red meat…and a limited amount of processed foods that are high in sugar, fat or additives.

Scientific evidence: Research has shown that people who consume more than four daily servings of vegetables have a 40% lower rate of cognitive decline than those who get less than one daily serving.

What I do: I try to eat more vegetables, particularly broccoli, cauliflower and other crucifers—there's strong evidence of their brain-protective effects.

Helpful: I'm not a veggie lover, so I roast vegetables with olive oil in the oven to make them more appetizing. Whenever possible, I use brain-healthy spices such as rosemary and turmeric.

STEP 3: **Guard your sleep.** During the day, harmful waste products accumulate in the brain. These wastes, including the amyloid protein that's linked to Alzheimer's, are mainly eliminated at night during deep (stages 3 and 4) sleep.

Scientific evidence: In a long-term Swedish study, men who reported poor sleep were 1.5 times more likely to develop Alzheimer's than those with better sleep.

Regardless of your age, you need a good night's sleep. While ideal sleep times vary depending on the person, sleeping less than six hours or more than nine hours nightly is linked to increased risk for cardiovascular disease—another Alzheimer's risk factor. If you don't feel rested when you wake up, talk to your doctor about your sleep quality.

What I do: I often take a 10-minute nap during the day. Brief naps (especially between 2 pm and 4 pm, which syncs with most people's circadian rhythms) can be restorative.

STEP 4: **Don't be a loner.** Having regular social interaction is strongly associated with healthy aging.

Scientific evidence: Older adults who frequently spend time with others—for example, sharing meals and volunteering—have about a 70% lower rate of cognitive decline than those who don't socialize much.

What I do: To stay socially active, I regularly Skype, attend conferences and stay in touch with other scientists and postdoc students.

If you're lonely, any form of social interaction is better than none. One study found that people who used computers regularly—to write e-mails, for example—were less lonely than those who didn't. If you can't connect in person, do a video chat or Facebook update at least once a day.

Also helpful: Having a pet. Pets are sometimes better listeners than spouses!

STEP 5: **Stay calm.** People who are often stressed are more likely to experience brain shrinkage.

Scientific evidence: In a three-year study of people with mild cognitive impairment (a condition that often precedes Alzheimer's), those with severe anxiety had a 135% increased risk for Alzheimer's, compared with those who were calmer.

What I do: I go for long walks.

Other great stress reducers: Having a positive mental attitude, deep breathing, yoga, tai chi, meditation—and even watching funny movies. Practice what works for you.

STEP 6: **Push yourself intellectually.** So-called "brain workouts" help prevent Alzheimer's—perhaps by increasing cognitive reserve (the stored memories/cognitive skills that you can draw on later in life)...and possibly by accelerating the growth of new brain cells.

Scientific evidence: In an important study, older adults (including those with a genetic risk factor for Alzheimer's) who frequently read, played board games or engaged in other mental activities were able to postpone the development of the disease by almost a decade.

But don't fool yourself—if you're an accomplished pianist, then banging out a tune won't help much even though a nonmusician is likely to benefit from learning to play. Push your mental abilities—do math problems in your head, memorize a poem, become a tutor, etc.

What I do: To challenge myself intellectually, I read novels and practice my foreign language skills—I do research in Latin America, so I work on my Spanish.

What You Don't Know About Preventing Alzheimer's

Dean Sherzai, MD, a neurologist and director of the Alzheimer's Disease Prevention Program at Cedars-Sinai Medical Center in Los Angeles.

Alzheimer's disease is hands-down one of the most feared diseases. But simply worrying that you'll develop the illness doesn't do any good. A far better approach is to take action—now!

What's new: Around the country, respected medical centers and hospitals are now creating Alzheimer's prevention programs staffed by neurologists and researchers who help people do all that they can do to avoid this devastating condition.*

Even if you're only in your 30s or 40s, it's wise to see a neurologist if you have a family history of Alzheimer's disease...or if, at any age, you're noticing mental changes (such as memory loss) that concern you. Everyone has momentary lapses—forgetting where you left your keys, for example—but those that impact your life, such as missing appointments, should be evaluated.

*To find an Alzheimer's prevention program near you, check with a local chapter of the Alzheimer's Association, ALZ.org, a local university or state or local agency for the aging.

What Can You Do?

An increasing number of Alzheimer's experts now believe that preventive lifestyle approaches may help preserve memory and cognitive abilities. It's best to start before any disease-related changes occur in the brain. By the time symptoms are recognizable, the disease already has a foothold and the benefits of intervention will be nominal. While you may think that you already know the main Alzheimer's prevention strategies, key recommendations include specifics that really make a difference. *Steps to take…*

•**Control your blood sugar.** Most Alzheimer's patients have higher-than-normal blood sugar levels or full-blown diabetes. In a study that tracked more than 2,000 patients for roughly seven years, those with a glucose reading of 115 mg/dL, on average, had an 18% higher risk for dementia than those with levels of 100 mg/dL or lower (normal range). The higher the blood sugar levels, the greater the Alzheimer's risk. It's not yet clear why elevated blood sugar increases cognitive risks, but it could be linked to the inflammation that accompanies blood glucose disorders.

Advice: Avoid simple carbohydrates such as white bread and white rice that cause blood sugar to spike. Also, emerging evidence shows that eating a lot of sugar may cause Alzheimer's brain changes—so avoid sugar.

Recommended: No more than nine teaspoons of added sugars for men each day…six teaspoons for women. This may sound like a lot, but it's actually a lot less than many people get. Added sugars are in many foods—not only in such things as sweetened yogurt and fruit drinks but also in pasta sauces, breads and salad dressings. Also, get screened for diabetes at three-year intervals, starting at age 45—sooner (and more frequently) if you have diabetes risk factors such as obesity and/or a family history.

•**Consume the "Big 3."** The Mediterranean diet, which includes fish, fruit, beans, vegetables, whole grains and monounsaturated fat (such as olive oil), has been widely promoted for brain health. But which specific foods are most likely to help keep you mentally sharp? *There's strong evidence for…*

•Fruit and vegetable juices, such as pomegranate, blueberry and grape. A nine-year study of 1,836 participants found that those who drank fruit or vegetable juices at least three times a week were 76% less likely to develop Alzheimer's than those who had them less than once a week.

Possible reason: Juices have a high concentration of anti-inflammatory antioxidants—and this may help interrupt some of the brain changes (such as beta-amyloid deposits) that occur in Alzheimer's patients. A daily serving of a juiced mixture of fresh vegetables and low-sugar fruits, such as berries, lime or cantaloupe, is a good source of antioxidants and nutrients. Fruits high in sugar, such as bananas and mangoes, should be avoided, since as mentioned earlier, recent research has linked higher sugar levels with cognitive decline and dementia.

•Fatty fish. Researchers recently announced that people with high blood levels of omega-3 fatty acids had increased volume in the hippocampus, a part of the brain that's affected in those with cognitive decline. Other research has shown that there's less Alzheimer's in parts of the world where people eat the most fish.

One problem is that people often eat the wrong kind of fish. It must be omega-3–rich, fatty fish.

Best choices: Salmon, herring, mackerel, sardines or tuna, eaten at least twice a week. If you don't like fish, you can take a daily supplement. Fish oil supplements approved by the FDA include Lovaza, Epanova and Omtryg. Because they are available by prescription, they may be covered by your insurance. Alternatively, you can take an over-the-counter fish oil supplement (check with your doctor first—fish oil can raise risk for bleeding). Flaxseed, chia seeds and walnuts contain a plant-based omega-3.

Fun Way to Boost Brain Health

Learn a new word every day! As people age, the brain relies on "cognitive reserve" (healthy neural networks) to compensate for loss of cognitive function such as memory. In a recent study of more than 300 people over age 50, healthy participants had a stronger vocabulary than those with mild cognitive impairment.

To keep your neural networks strong: Play daily word games, or sign up for Word of the Day apps.

Cristina Lojo Seoane, PhD, researcher, department of developmental psychology, University of Santiago de Compostela, Spain.

•Vegetables—and more vegetables. With all the focus on brain-healthy fruits such as blueberries, vegetables are often forgotten. That's a mistake. In a study of more than 3,700 people, those who consumed the most vegetables (a median of 4.1 daily servings) had 38% less cognitive decline than those who ate the least. Good choices for those four or more daily servings are kale, spinach, brussels sprouts, broccoli and red bell peppers.

•**Give your mind the right kind of workout.** Crosswords and Sudoku help but less than you might think. They get easy with practice and target only some parts of the brain.

Better: Activities that challenge your brain on multiple levels—and stay challenging no matter how long you do them.

Examples: Playing a musical instrument, painting and even playing some challenging video or board games.

Also: Look for hobbies that use the hands and the mind—they require focus, memory, problem-solving, spatial visualization and other skills.

Advice: List 10 activities that you enjoy, and try to do three or four of them daily. If one activity doesn't stimulate a part of your brain, another probably will.

•**Get more exercise—safely.** When it comes to preserving brain health, nothing beats exercise. It improves circulation and increases the amounts of glucose and oxygen that reach the brain.

Advice: Be sure to exercise safely. An injury will deprive you of one of your strongest defenses against Alzheimer's. Outdoor exercise can increase risk for falls and other injuries. If you're not that sure-footed, go for indoor exercise using a machine such as a recumbent bicycle or elliptical trainer. Otherwise, take brisk walks outdoors. Aim for 30 minutes of moderate-to-vigorous exercise (breathing hard and fast with increased heart rate) on most days of the week, plus strength, flexibility and balance-improving activities. (Start with five-minute sessions if you're not used to it.)

A Medication Worth Trying?

High blood pressure is widely known to increase Alzheimer's risk. What you may not realize is that the type of medicine used to control high blood pressure could also affect your Alzheimer's risk.

Interesting finding: When the medical records of more than five million patients were reviewed, those who took blood pressure drugs called angiotensin II receptor blockers (ARBs), such as *irbesartan* (Avapro), *losartan* (Cozaar) and *azilsartan* (Edarbi), had a 35% to 40% lower risk of developing Alzheimer's or other brain diseases than those prescribed other blood pressure drugs. What makes these drugs different? It's possible that blocking the renin-angiotensin system provides neurological benefits in addition to lowering blood pressure.

The research is not definitive, so your doctor won't prescribe an ARB just to prevent Alzheimer's disease. But if you're already taking blood pressure medication, you may want to ask about trying an ARB.

Five Surprising Ways to Prevent Alzheimer's ... # 1: Check Your Tap Water

Marwan Sabbagh, MD, neurologist, and director of the Alzheimer's disease and memory disorders division at Barrow Neurological Institute at Dignity Health St. Joseph's Hospital and Medical Center, Phoenix, Arizona. He is author of *The Alzheimer's Prevention Cookbook: 100 Recipes to Boost Brain Health.* MarwanSabbaghMD.com

Every 68 seconds, another American develops Alzheimer's disease, the fatal brain disease that steals memory and personality. It's the fifth-leading cause of death among people age 65 and older.

You can lower your likelihood of getting Alzheimer's disease by reducing controllable and well-known risk factors. *But new scientific research reveals that there are also little-known "secret" risk factors that you can address...*

Copper in Tap Water

A scientific paper published in *Journal of Trace Elements in Medicine and Biology* theorizes that inorganic copper found in nutritional supplements and in drinking water is an important factor in today's Alzheimer's epidemic.

Science has established that amyloid-beta plaques—inflammation-causing cellular debris found in the brains of people with Alzheimer's—contain high levels of copper. Animal research shows that small amounts of inorganic copper in drinking water worsen Alzheimer's. Studies on people have linked the combination of copper and a high-fat diet to memory loss and mental decline. It may be that copper sparks amyloid-beta plaques to generate more oxidation and inflammation, further injuring brain cells.

What to do: There is plenty of copper in our diets—no one needs additional copper from a multivitamin/mineral supplement. Look for a supplement with no copper or a minimal amount (500 micrograms).

I also recommend filtering water. Water-filter pitchers, such as ones by Brita, can reduce the presence of copper. I installed a reverse-osmosis water filter in my home a few years ago when the evidence for the role of copper in Alzheimer's became compelling.

Vitamin D Deficiency

Mounting evidence shows that a low blood level of vitamin D may increase Alzheimer's risk.

A study in *Journal of Alzheimer's Disease* analyzed 10 studies exploring the link between vitamin D and Alzheimer's. Researchers found that low blood levels of vitamin D were linked to a 40% increased risk for Alzheimer's.

The researchers from UCLA, also writing in *Journal of Alzheimer's Disease*, theorize that vitamin D may protect the brain by reducing amyloid-beta and inflammation.

What to do: The best way to make sure that your blood level of vitamin D is protective is to ask your doctor to test it—and then, if needed, to help you correct your level to greater than 60 nanograms per milliliter (ng/mL). That correction may require 1,000 IU to 2,000 IU of vitamin D daily...or another individualized supplementation strategy.

Important: When your level is tested, make sure that it is the 25-hydroxyvitamin D, or 25(OH)D, test and not the 1.25-dihydroxy-vitamin D test. The latter test does not accurately measure blood levels of vitamin D but is sometimes incorrectly ordered. Also, ask for your exact numerical results. Levels above 30 ng/mL are considered "normal," but in my view, the 60 ng/mL level is the minimum that is protective.

Hormone Replacement Therapy After Menopause

Research shows that starting hormone-replacement therapy (HRT) within five years of entering menopause and using hormones for 10 or more years reduces the risk for Alzheimer's by 30%. But an 11-year study of 1,768 women, published in *Neurology*, shows that those who started a combination of estrogen-progestin therapy five years or more after the onset of menopause had a 93% higher risk for Alzheimer's.

What to do: If you are thinking about initiating hormone-replacement therapy five years or more after the onset of menopause, talk to your doctor about the possible benefits and risks.

A Concussion

A study published in *Neurology* showed that NFL football players had nearly four times higher risk for Alzheimer's than the general population—no doubt from repeated brain injuries incurred while playing football.

Control Your Alzheimer's Risk

Many of the biggest risk factors for Alzheimer's disease are modifiable—lack of physical activity, depression, smoking, midlife hypertension, midlife obesity and diabetes. Changing or eliminating these risks could potentially prevent 2.9 million Alzheimer's cases in the US.

Deborah Barnes, PhD, MPH, associate professor of psychiatry, University of California, San Francisco, and leader of a comprehensive review published online in *The Lancet Neurology*.

What most people don't realize: Your risk of developing Alzheimer's is doubled if you've ever had a serious concussion that resulted in loss of consciousness—this newer evidence shows that it is crucially important to prevent head injuries of any kind throughout your life.

What to do: Fall-proof your home, with commonsense measures such as adequate lighting, eliminating or securing throw rugs and keeping stairways clear. Wear shoes with firm soles and low heels, which also helps prevent falls.

If you've ever had a concussion, it's important to implement the full range of Alzheimer's-prevention strategies in this article.

Not Having a Purpose in Life

In a seven-year study published in *Archives of General Psychiatry*, researchers at the Rush Alzheimer's Disease Center in Chicago found that people who had a "purpose in life" were 2.4 times less likely to develop Alzheimer's.

What to do: The researchers found that the people who agreed with the following statements were less likely to develop Alzheimer's and mild cognitive impairment—"I feel good when I think of what I have done in the past and what I hope to do in the future" and "I have a sense of direction and purpose in life."

If you cannot genuinely agree with the above statements, there are things you can do to change that—in fact, you even can change the way you feel about your past. It takes a bit of resolve…some action…and perhaps help from a qualified mental health counselor.

One way to start: Think about and make a list of some activities that would make your life more meaningful. Ask yourself, *Am I doing these?*…and then write down small, realistic goals that will involve you more in those activities, such as volunteering one hour every week at a local hospital or signing up for a class at your community college next semester.

The following steps are crucial in the fight against Alzheimer's disease…

- **Lose weight if you're overweight.**
- **Control high blood pressure.**
- **Exercise regularly.**
- **Engage in activities that challenge your mind.**
- **Eat a diet rich in colorful fruits and vegetables** and low in saturated fat, such as the Mediterranean diet.
- **Take a daily supplement** containing 2,000 milligrams of omega-3 fatty acids.

How to Cut Your Risk for Alzheimer's...by Half

Majid Fotuhi, MD, PhD, neurologist, medical director of the NeuroGrow Brain Fitness Center in McLean, Virginia, and affiliate staff at Johns Hopkins Medicine, Baltimore. He is also author of *The Memory Cure* and coauthor of *The New York Times Crosswords to Keep Your Brain Young.*

The prevalence of memory and thinking problems—including Alzheimer's disease and other forms of dementia—declined in the US by nearly 30% during a recent nine-year period.

Why did this happen? Partly because many adults are doing a better job at controlling significant dementia risk factors, including blood pressure (below 120/80 mm Hg is optimal) and cholesterol (below 200 mg/dL is the target for most people's total cholesterol).

But there are other strategies to reduce dementia risk even further. Although some vulnerability to Alzheimer's and other forms of dementia can be genetic, an ever-increasing body of evidence shows that adopting a healthful lifestyle often can cut a person's risk by half. *What you need to know...*

Overlooked Risk Factors

Dementia occurs when brain cells are progressively damaged by excessive accumulation of proteins, such as amyloid. These proteins trigger inflammation, causing more damage to nearby brain cells. But that's not the only trigger. The brain needs a constant supply of oxygen, hormones and nutrients such as blood sugar (glucose). Interruptions in the supply—due to narrowed and blocked blood vessels, multiple small strokes that may pass unnoticed and even heart failure, kidney disease and chronic lung disease—can kill brain cells.

Other dementia risk factors that are sometimes overlooked...

•**Belly fat.** Abdominal fat is strongly linked to an increased risk for heart disease, and two recent studies have shown an association between belly fat and dementia.

Evidence: A study of more than 6,500 men and women, published in *Neurology*, found that those with the most belly fat during their 40s were nearly three times as likely to develop dementia over the next 30 to 40 years, compared with those who had the least belly fat.

Alzheimer's prevention step: Regardless of your age, strive for a fit body. Your waist measurement in inches should be no more than half your height, in inches.

•**Diabetes.** Research supports a link between diabetes and dementia. One Swedish study of 2,269 men found that those whose secretion of the hormone insulin was low in response to glucose at age 50 (a sign of impaired glucose metabolism that is likely to progress to diabetes) were significantly more likely to develop dementia over the next 32 years.

Alzheimer's prevention step: Your blood glucose level after fasting overnight should be less than 100 mg/dL. People with levels of 100 mg/dL to 125 mg/dL may be at risk for diabetes and should be closely monitored by their physicians. Levels of 126 mg/dL and higher indicate diabetes. Follow your doctor's advice on the frequency of fasting blood-glucose testing.

•**Smoking and heavy drinking.** People with a history of smoking or heavy drinking appear to develop Alzheimer's sooner than others.

Evidence: In a Florida study of nearly 1,000 people diagnosed with Alzheimer's, those who smoked more than a pack per day developed Alzheimer's 2.3 years before those who were not heavy smokers. Those who drank more than two drinks per day developed it 4.8 years earlier than those who drank less.

Alzheimer's prevention step: If you smoke, quit now. If you drink, ask your doctor whether moderate drinking is beneficial for you. Moderate alcohol consumption has been shown in some studies to help prevent cognitive decline. Women should not exceed one drink (wine, beer or hard liquor) daily...men, no more than two drinks daily.

Exercise Really Does Help

Even if you're aware that exercise helps protect against dementia, few people realize just how important it is. Besides maintaining good circulation to ensure a steady supply of nutrients and oxygen to the brain, physical activity increases production of brain-derived neurotrophic factor—a protein that triggers brain cell growth.

Evidence: Sedentary retirees started walking three times a week. Six months later, their brains—as measured by magnetic resonance imaging (MRI) scans—had grown by 3%, on average, roughly the equivalent of taking three years off the age of their brains.

Alzheimer's prevention step: Get at least 30 minutes of moderate exercise (such as brisk walking) most days of the week. If you don't like walking, try dancing, cycling or golf. Any physical activity is better than nothing—and the more, the better.

Get the Right Brain Foods

Foods that help protect your brain...

•**Omega-3 fatty acids** are the most abundant of the polyunsaturated fatty acids that comprise up to 20% of the brain's volume. Some people get their omega-3s from fish-oil capsules—which contain both *eicosapentaenoic acid* (EPA) and *docosahexaenoic acid* (DHA). DHA is the most important for brain health and is recommended (along with EPA) for heart health by the American Heart Association.

Alzheimer's prevention step: Ask your doctor about taking an omega-3 supplement that contains at least 400 mg of DHA per daily dose. Or eat two to three servings of cold-water fish (such as wild salmon, mackerel and sardines) weekly.

•**Antioxidants protect the brain against cumulative damage caused by highly reactive chemicals known as "free radicals."** An eight-year study of 5,000 people identified vitamins E and C as particularly important for brain health.

> ### Even Slightly High Blood Sugar Hurts Memory
>
> People with blood sugar at the high end of the normal range performed worse on a memory test than people with lower blood sugar levels.
>
> *Also:* People with high blood sugar had a smaller hippocampus, the area of the brain that plays a crucial role in memory and spatial navigation.
>
> *Best:* Get your blood sugar level checked regularly...monitor your diet...and exercise to keep your blood sugar levels low.
>
> Study of 141 people, average age 63, by researchers at Charité-Medical University of Berlin, Germany, published in Neurology.

Alzheimer's prevention step: Whenever possible, get your vitamins E and C from fruits and vegetables—this also will increase your intake of other powerful antioxidants. Kiwifruit, papaya and pomegranates are particularly good sources. Aim for four to five servings daily of fruits and vegetables. If you prefer a supplement, take 300 international units (IU) of vitamin E and 500 mg of vitamin C daily.

•**Curcumin is the yellow pigment of turmeric, the primary ingredient in curry powder.** Laboratory tests have shown that curcumin helps dissolve the abnormal amyloid formations of Alzheimer's disease.

Alzheimer's prevention step: Cook with curcumin (try it in curried chicken, soups and vegetables) or take a 200-mg supplement daily.

Also helpful: A regular regimen of "brain fitness" activities.

Memory Self-Test

Questions to ask yourself...

1. Have you ever gotten lost when you drive home?

2. **Have you forgotten being at major appointments or events?** Forgetting names of people you met at a recent party is not cause for concern, but forgetting that you attended the party could signal a possible memory problem.

3. **Has anyone around you complained that you tend to repeat the same questions four or five times?**

4. **Have you stopped any of your hobbies or routines because of memory problems?**

5. **Have you reduced your work responsibilities or hours mainly due to poor memory?** For example, did you take early retirement because you can't keep up with the same work you've done for years?

If you answered "yes" to any of these questions, speak to your doctor about getting a neurological evaluation.

Bad Vision Boosts Alzheimer's Risk

Mary A.M. Rogers, PhD, research associate professor, department of internal medicine, University of Michigan, and research director of the Patient Safety Enhancement Program, University of Michigan Health System, Ann Arbor.

Want to give yourself a better chance of evading Alzheimer's disease? Get your eyes checked. Recent research reveals that treating vision problems can actually reduce the risk for dementia, including Alzheimer's disease.

Seeds for this study were planted with information from the Aging, Demographics, and Memory Study, when University of Michigan researchers noticed that people with dementia tended to have had fewer eye procedures prior to their diagnoses than those without dementia. *This led the team to ask two questions...*

•**Does poor vision contribute to the development of dementia?**

•**Does treating visual disorders reduce the likelihood of developing dementia?**

Can You See Dementia in Your Future?

Using data from Medicare and the nationally representative Health and Retirement Study, the Michigan researchers followed 625 elderly Americans (none of whom had dementia at the outset) for an average of 10 years. Based on a scale that ranked vision from excellent (one) to totally blind (six), they found that the risk for dementia increased 52%, on average, with each step up the scale. The study results suggest that the problems with declining vision preceded the dementia. This is thought to be the first epidemiologic study that points to treatment of vision problems as being protective against the development of late-life dementia.

Some of the connections between poor vision and dementia symptoms seem obvious, while others are not yet understood. For instance, people with poor vision may be less likely to participate in the kinds of activities, such as reading, playing board games and engaging in physical activities, that can be protective against cognitive decline. Other research indicates that visual loss can lead to structural changes in the brain, but notes that more studies are needed to understand why.

See Your Doctor!

Good news came out of this study too. When elderly people received appropriate treatment for their visual difficulties—which can include procedures such as corneal transplant, cataract removal and lens insertion, and treatment for retinal detachment, lesions and other eye disorders—their probability of developing dementia decreased. Even one visit to an ophthalmologist was associated with a lower risk.

It is wise to visit your doctor if you are having any vision problems—it may improve your health and your life in several important ways.

What's Your Real Risk for Alzheimer's?

Gayatri Devi, MD, director of New York Memory and Healthy Aging Services and an attending physician at Lenox Hill Hospital, both in New York City, and clinical professor of neurology at SUNY Downstate Medical Center in Brooklyn. A board-certified neurologist, Dr. Devi is author of *The Spectrum of Hope: An Optimistic and New Approach to Alzheimer's Disease.* NYBrain.org

Older adults fear Alzheimer's disease more than cancer. But how worried do you really need to be?

Let's start with the good news...if you have a first-degree relative with the disease (a parent or sibling), you're only at a slightly greater risk than someone who does not have a first-degree relative with Alzheimer's. That's because there are many factors that affect your risk for Alzheimer's...not just your genes (more on this later).

Poor lifestyle choices (such as an unhealthy diet and/or not exercising regularly) also increase your risk—much more so than genetics. That's why one twin in a set of identical twins can get Alzheimer's while the other twin stays healthy.

There's even more good news—a diagnosis of Alzheimer's is not necessarily the disaster you probably imagine it to be. Alzheimer's is now viewed by most medical professionals as a so-called "spectrum disorder," rather than a single disease, because different people have different symptoms and different rates of progression.

Most people diagnosed with Alzheimer's are not on the catastrophic end of that spectrum—they are not going to forget who they are or the names of their loved ones. Most will live at home and die at home, particularly if the disease is detected early and symptoms are well-managed with treatments such as medication, a healthy diet and regular exercise.

Bottom line: Even if you are at genetic risk, you can use lifestyle modifications to reduce your risk to below that of someone who has no family history of Alzheimer's.

How to Tweak Your Lifestyle

Most cases of late-onset Alzheimer's disease are preventable—with simple lifestyle changes that reduce one's risk for the disease.

The brain changes of Alzheimer's (the so-called plaques and tangles, which are accumulations of toxic proteins) can start 20 to 30 years before the onset of symptoms. But research shows that preventive measures can stop plaques and tangles as well as symptoms from ever developing...and even prevent symptoms if your brain is riddled with plaques and tangles.

Factors that increase Alzheimer's risk for everyone—regardless of one's genetic predisposition—and how to counteract them...

•**Sedentary lifestyle.** Exercising for 45 minutes, at least three days a week (at an intensity that is 50% higher than your resting heart rate) is a must for reducing your risk for Alzheimer's. It stimulates blood flow to the brain, allowing new neurons to grow. Research shows that it decreases your risk for Alzheimer's by 40%.

Surprising fact: Cognitive abilities such as memory improve by 10% immediately after exercise.

•**Poor diet.** A diet loaded with saturated fats, refined sugar and processed foods increases the risk for Alzheimer's. A Mediterranean-style diet—rich in whole foods such as vegetables, fruits, beans, whole grains and fish—is proven to reduce the risk for Alzheimer's by 50%.

Also helpful: A healthy breakfast, which consists of protein, fiber and fruit. Research shows that if you take in less than 7% of your daily calories at breakfast, your risk for heart disease and Alzheimer's more than doubles.

•**Limited mental stimulation.** Regular mental stimulation reduces Alzheimer's risk—in fact, research shows that even reading a newspaper every day can help prevent the disease.

Best: Engage in a type of mental stimulation that is different from what you do at work, thereby stimulating a different part of your brain.

Example: If you are a computer programmer, learn how to play golf.

•**Social isolation.** Healthy social relationships—with family, friends and in the community—decrease the risk for Alzheimer's disease. Feeling lonely doubles the risk…living alone raises it fivefold.

•**Heart disease.** Circulatory problems cause heart disease and Alzheimer's disease. Medical and lifestyle treatments for cardiovascular issues, including high blood pressure, reduce Alzheimer's risk.

Bottom line: What's good for your heart is good for your brain.

•**Diabetes.** Some experts label Alzheimer's "type 3 diabetes" because of the established link between chronically high blood sugar and the risk for Alzheimer's disease—a person with diabetes has a 57% higher risk of developing the disease. Controlling high blood sugar with medical and lifestyle treatments is crucial for reducing Alzheimer's risk.

Helpful: Keep your glucose level below 100 mg/dL.

•**Insomnia.** Poor sleep increases risk for Alzheimer's, probably because brain plaque is cleared most effectively during sleep. But sleep medications aren't the answer—they also interfere with the clearance of brain plaque. What works better: Good sleep hygiene, such as going to bed and waking up at the same time every day.

Also helpful: Don't work on your computer in bed or keep your cell phone on your bedside table.

What's Your Genetic Risk?

Genetics is a strong factor when Alzheimer's begins at a young age. The early-onset form is an aggressive familial illness that can occur, in extremely rare cases, as early as in one's 20s, with most people developing the disease in their 50s or 60s. The child of a parent with early-onset Alzheimer's has a 50% chance of developing the disease. Fortunately, early-onset constitutes only 5% of all cases of Alzheimer's disease.

On the other hand, most cases of late-onset Alzheimer's (beginning after age 65) are not inherited. Instead, many medical and lifestyle factors contribute to the development of the illness.

Compelling scientific research: In one of the largest scientific studies that I have ever completed, published in *Archives of Neurology*, I looked at more than 5,500 siblings and parents of patients with Alzheimer's—alongside age-matched adults who did not have the disease.

Presuming (for uniform statistical analysis) that everyone in the study lived to age 90, I found that those with a first-degree relative with Alzheimer's had about a one-in-four chance of developing late-onset Alzheimer's—whereas those without an afflicted relative had a one-in-five chance of doing so.

In other words, if neither your parents nor siblings have (or had) Alzheimer's (and you live to age 90), you still have a 20% chance of getting the disease—while a person whose parent or sibling had Alzheimer's has a 26% chance.

Takeaway: Having a parent or sibling with Alzheimer's puts you at a relatively small increased risk for the disease. Exception: A person with late-onset Alzheimer's who also has a variant of the apolipoprotein E gene—APOE e4 (the most damaging of the so-called "Alzheimer's genes")—is more likely to have rapid progression of the disease.

Genetic Testing

My take on genetic testing for Alzheimer's: It may be appropriate only for people with a family history of early-onset Alzheimer's disease (before age 65). If a parent has early-onset Alzheimer's, as mentioned earlier, the child has a 50% chance of developing the disease. An estimated 200,000 Americans have the early-onset form of the disease.

If you have this type of family history, consult your doctor and a genetic counselor about genetic testing. Not all the genes that trigger early-onset Alzheimer's are known, but some are. If you decide to have a genetic test—and the test finds that you have one of the genetic mutations for Alzheimer's—you and your family can take that fact into account in various ways.

For example, you would want to create a step-by-step action plan for dealing with the disease, even before symptoms develop, by preparing for the future with advanced directives and financial planning...and perhaps consider entering one of the clinical trials that are testing new drugs to slow Alzheimer's development. (To find such a trial, consult ClinicalTrials.gov and search "early-onset Alzheimer's.")

Important: If you don't have a family history of early-onset Alzheimer's, I typically do not recommend genetic testing. The results would not accurately quantify your risk, and it's crucial that you implement key medical treatments (such as those for high blood pressure or diabetes) and lifestyle changes to reduce your risk for Alzheimer's whether or not you have a genetic variant for late-onset Alzheimer's.

Having a Purpose in Life Prevents Dementia

Patricia A. Boyle, PhD, neuropsychologist, Rush Alzheimer's Disease Center, and associate professor, department of behavioral sciences, Rush University Medical Center, both in Chicago. Her study was published in *Archives of General Psychiatry*.

You already know that staying physically and mentally active may help stave off dementia, but researchers have found yet another protective trick—having a purpose in life.

The study analyzed 246 senior citizens who received annual cognitive testing for about 10 years. Each was asked questions to determine whether he or she had a strong purpose in life. When participants died, they underwent brain autopsies.

What the researchers found was that in participants who had a lot of plaques and tangles in their brains—abnormal structures in and around the brain's nerve cells that are hallmarks of Alzheimer's disease—the rate of cognitive decline had been about 30% slower for people who had a strong purpose in life compared with those who had a weaker purpose or no purpose at all.

Here's a possible explanation: The stronger your purpose in life, the less likely you'll suffer cognitive decline as you age, even if your brain is affected by Alzheimer's signs.

Social Connections Prevent Memory Loss

A recent study of more than 16,000 people age 50 and older asked participants to take verbal memory tests over six years.

Findings: Those who had the fewest social connections with friends, family and in the community suffered decline in memory capacity at twice the rate as those with the most.

Conclusion: This is another example of how being socially engaged is beneficial for mental health.

Lisa F. Berkman, PhD, department of Sociology, Human Development and Health, Harvard School of Public Health, lead study author.

This might mean that you can preserve your cognitive ability by making sure that you have a purpose.

Of course, it could be the other way around—it could be that some people have a biological problem that makes them less able to cope with brain plaques and tangles and, also, less able to feel that their lives have purpose.

Go for It Anyway

The study doesn't prove whether purposefulness helps our brains work better or is simply a side effect of a brain that is already working better. Maybe research will determine that one day. But on the other hand, since having a sense of purpose seems to make people happier, why not cultivate one?

The study subject's life purpose is defined as "the sense that one's life has meaning and direction—that one is intentional and motivated to engage in activities that one finds important and fulfilling." In other words, it's what gets you out of bed each day and makes you feel that life is worth living.

A purpose doesn't have to be ambitious or complicated. In fact, many purposes are simple. It just can't have a definite end point—it has to last throughout your life. For example, some purposes include spending time every day with loved ones...helping other people (for example through long-term volunteer work)...learning something new every day...or passing down a certain set of knowledge or skills to a younger generation. If you love running marathons or writing novels, make sure that your goal is to continue pursuing those goals through life—and not just run one marathon or write one novel.

It's not so much what your purpose is—what's critical is how it makes you feel. If it stirs you up inside and makes you feel passionate, energetic and excited, then you've found it!

Get These Minerals Out of Your Brain!

Neal D. Barnard, MD, president of the nonprofit Physicians Committee for Responsible Medicine. He is author of *Power Foods for the Brain: An Effective 3-Step Plan to Protect Your Mind and Strengthen Your Memory*. PCRM.org

Chances are you're doing everything that you can to eat plenty of "superfoods"—blueberries, walnuts and other nutritious and antioxidant-rich wonders—that many scientists believe help reduce risk for a variety of chronic health problems, including Alzheimer's disease.

The missing part of the story: What you may not know is that most people get too much of certain nutrients—even those found in some superfoods—that have long been considered an important part of a nutritious diet.

Iron, copper and zinc, which are widely recognized as key nutrients, actually are metallic minerals. They are common in many of the foods you may be eating, the water you drink—and even in some of the supplements you may be taking to improve your health.

What researchers are now discovering: Excessive amounts of iron, copper and zinc can produce free radicals that impair memory.

In fact, scientists have discovered that these metals are more prevalent in the brains of Alzheimer's patients than in people without the disease. Even in healthy adults, high levels appear to interfere with normal brain functions.

> **To Protect Your Brain: Hold Off on Retirement**
>
> Delaying retirement may protect your brain. For each additional year that a person worked before retiring, dementia risk dropped by 3% in a recent analysis. That means someone who retired at age 60 had a 15% greater chance of developing dementia, on average, than someone who retired at 65.
>
> *Theory:* The mental stimulation and social connections at work may keep the brain healthy.
>
> Analysis of the records of more than 400,000 retired workers in France by researchers at National Institute of Health and Medical Research, Paris, presented at the 2013 Alzheimer's Association International Conference.

Three Newly Discovered Dangers

Your body does need iron, copper and zinc, but only in miniscule amounts. If you exceed these levels, your brain is at risk. *What to watch out for…*

•**Iron.** Unless you have been diagnosed with a condition that requires supplemental iron, such as anemia, you probably don't need more than you're already getting from your diet—and even that might be too much.

Compelling evidence: In a study of 793 adults, those who had the most iron in their blood did worse on cognitive tests than those with normal levels.

In a study of 881 adults, those with high hemoglobin levels (a measure of iron in the blood) were three times more likely to develop Alzheimer's disease than those with normal levels. Hemoglobin levels above 13.7 g/dL were associated with increased Alzheimer's risk. Those whose iron levels are too low are also at risk for Alzheimer's.

My advice: Emphasize plant-based foods in your diet. These foods can contain as much iron as what's found in meat—but our bodies are better able to regulate our intake of the type of iron found in plant-based foods, such as spinach, dried apricots, lima beans and wheat germ. Your body absorbs more of this nonheme iron when you need it and absorbs less when you don't.

In contrast, the heme iron in meats, poultry, fish and shellfish (particularly oysters) is absorbed whether you need it or not. Because of this, a high-meat diet is a main cause of iron overload, which potentially damages not only your brain but also your heart.

Other smart steps…

•**Don't use iron cookware.** A significant amount of iron leaches from uncoated cast-iron pots, pans and skillets into foods—particularly acidic foods, such as tomatoes.

•**Choose an iron-free product if you take a daily multisupplement.**

•**Read cereal labels.** Many breakfast cereals are fortified with iron. You don't need it.

Amount of iron you need in your diet: 8 mg per day for men age 19 and older and women age 51 and older. Women age 19 to 50 need 18 mg per day. (In general, women should get the lower amount of iron when they stop menstruating.)

•**Copper.** At proper levels, copper is essential for enzyme function and helps promote heart health and bone strength. At excess levels, copper—like iron—triggers the production of free radicals that can damage brain cells.

Important finding: A study of 1,451 people in southern California found that those who had the least copper in their blood were mentally sharper and had fewer problems with long- and short-term memory than those whose levels were high.

How copper may promote almost 20 years of aging: When high copper levels are combined with excess saturated fat in the diet—another risk factor for brain problems—the effect is particularly detrimental. Data from the Chicago Health and Aging Project found that high copper/saturated fat caused a loss of mental function that was the equivalent of 19 years of aging.

My advice: Don't take any supplement that contains copper. If you have copper plumbing, it's fine to use tap water for doing dishes and washing but not for cooking or drinking. It is better to use bottled water or water filtered with an activated carbon filter (such as those found in Brita pitchers).

You are unlikely to get too much copper from plant foods that are rich in the mineral such as whole grains, nuts and beans because they also contain natural compounds called phytates that limit copper absorption.

Amount of copper you need: 0.9 mg daily.

•**Zinc.** Our bodies need adequate zinc levels for key functions such as immunity, skin health and sexual function. Excessive amounts, however, are thought to promote the clumping of beta-amyloid proteins in the brain—the hallmark of Alzheimer's disease.

Much of the excess zinc in the American diet comes from supplements. If you take a multivitamin-mineral supplement and also eat fortified cereals or other foods that include zinc, such as oysters, pumpkin seeds or cocoa, you could be getting too much.

Amount of zinc you need: 11 mg daily for men and 8 mg for women.

Takeaway on Minerals

Testing is not needed to check levels of iron, copper and zinc in your blood. It is wise to simply avoid the mineral sources in this article. If you are getting too much of these minerals, your levels will gradually decline when you avoid excessive intakes.

Important: Avoid multivitamin-mineral supplements.

Better choices: "Vitamin only" supplements such as No Minerals Multivitamin by Nature's Blend or Vitamins Only by Solgar.

What About Aluminum?

This ubiquitous metal has never been considered a nutrient—it plays no role in the body. While questions have persisted for several years about whether aluminum interferes with brain health, recent studies suggest that the risk is real.

In the UK, researchers found that Alzheimer's cases occurred 50% more often in counties with high aluminum levels in the water. Other studies have had similar results.

My advice: While researchers search for definitive findings on aluminum, err on the side of caution...

•**Don't buy foods that contain aluminum.** Check food labels. Cheese products (such as the cheese on frozen pizza) often

Distrust Harms the Brain

People who habitually distrust others, believing that others act mainly in their own self-interest, are three times more likely to develop dementia than those who do not. That was the finding of a recent eight-year study of older adults (average age 71).

Why: Chronic negative emotions can impair cognitive function.

Possible explanation: Unstable blood pressure can disrupt blood flow to the brain, which could lead to dementia over time.

Anna-Maija Tolppanen, PhD, development director of neurology, University of Eastern Finland, Kuopio.

contain aluminum. So do baking powders and the baked goods that include them. You can buy an aluminum-free baking powder, such as the Rumford brand.

•**Don't take aluminum antacids.** Use an aluminum-free product, such as Tums. Other drugs, such as buffered aspirin, may also contain aluminum. Check the label.

•**Cook with steel-clad or porcelain-coated pots**…use wax paper instead of aluminum foil…and don't consume foods or beverages that come in aluminum cans.

•**Check your tap water.** If it's high in aluminum or other metals, use bottled water or a reverse osmosis filter. For more information about testing your water, visit the Environmental Protection Agency (EPA) website EPA.gov/ground-water-and-drinking-water. You can use the EPA website, cfpub.EPA.gov/safewater/ccr, to get information about the water sources in your area.

•**Avoid antiperspirants with aluminum.** Labels may say aluminum or alum to indicate an aluminum-containing ingredient.

Cholesterol Affects Future Dementia Risk

Rachel Whitmer, PhD, research scientist and epidemiologist in the division of research at Kaiser Permanente in Oakland, California, and senior author of a study of 9,844 people.

Sometimes it feels like developing dementia as we age is inevitable. But a recent large-scale, long-term study lends support to one risk-reduction strategy over which we do have significant control—cholesterol levels.

What this study found: Compared to people with normal cholesterol levels, those who had borderline-high cholesterol (200 mg/dL to 239 mg/dL) at age 40 to 45 were 52% more likely to develop dementia within 40 years. For those who had high cholesterol (240 mg/dL or above) at midlife, dementia risk was elevated 66%.

Lesson: What's good for the heart is good for the brain—so no matter what your age, if you have high cholesterol, talk to your doctor about cholesterol-reducing strategies, such as dietary changes, exercise and, if necessary, medication.

Watch for Anemia to Avoid Dementia

Study titled "Anemia and risk of dementia in older adults: Findings from the Health ABC study," published in *Neurology*.

Anemia—a shortage of oxygen-carrying red blood cells—is fairly common in older adults, affecting up to 24% of people age 65 and older. Meanwhile, Alzheimer's disease, the most common form of dementia, affects 15% of people age 65 to 74 and 44% of people age 75 to 84. And now studies have shown a link between the two disorders, and that's good news. Looking out for and addressing one (anemia) may have a strong impact on avoiding the other (dementia).

In one small study, the risk of dementia doubled within three years of an anemia diagnosis and, in another, anemia was associated with a 60% increased risk of Alzheimer's disease within 3.3 years. But while small studies are all well and fine to get a glimpse into new ways of seeing health problems, larger studies are needed to really make a strong case. And that's what an international team of researchers has done.

The team followed 2,552 people, age 70 to 79, who participated in an 11-year study called Health, Aging and Body Composition. Over the course of the study period, all of the participants were given memory tests to check for signs of dementia and blood tests for anemia. None of them had dementia at the start of the study, and 15% of them had anemia. By the end of the study, 18% of participants had Alzheimer's or another form of dementia. When the researchers compared rates of dementia between people who had or didn't have anemia, they discovered that having anemia was associated with a 41% higher risk for Alzheimer's or another form of dementia.

What to Do

How anemia is linked to dementia is not completely understood. Possible factors include simply being in poor health, not getting enough oxygen to the brain (those red blood cells!) or having an iron or vitamin B-12 deficiency. Whatever the connection, in case it is anemia that is actually causing dementia, you'll want to do whatever you can to recognize and treat the symptoms of anemia—and, of course, prevent anemia from ever happening in the first place.

Signs of anemia can be subtle at first and include fatigue, weakness, pale skin, fast or irregular heartbeat, trouble breathing, chest pain, trouble with memory and concentration, cold hands and feet and headache. So if you've been feeling fatigued and don't know why or have other symptoms just mentioned, make an appointment with your doctor, who will order a blood test to check for anemia.

If anemia is found, additional tests will be done to find the exact cause, and the results will determine treatment.

Although rare or hereditary forms of anemia require blood transfusions, others are corrected by treating the underlying cause, whether it be loss of blood from a bleeding ulcer or complications from an infection or a medication side effect. Fortunately, the most common form of anemia—that caused by an iron or B-12 deficiency—is managed with good nutrition and vitamin and mineral supplements. It might be a simple correction that lets you avoid a horrific outcome.

Preventing Anemia

Since prevention is best, keep your diet rich in iron, folate, vitamin B-12, and vitamin C (which is essential for iron absorption). Foods that will give you the iron you need include red meat, beans, dried fruit, and green leafy vegetables, such as spinach. Besides vitamin C, citrus fruits provide folate. Other good sources of folate include green leafy veggies, beans and bananas. As for vitamin B-12, rely on salmon, shellfish, beef and dairy. And if you are vegan or vegetarian (or have a large B-12 deficiency), you likely already know that you need to get B-12 from supplementation.

The Truth About Weight and Dementia

Deborah Gustafson, PhD, professor of neurology, SUNY Downstate Medical Center, Brooklyn, New York. Her review, titled "2003-2013: a decade of body mass index, Alzheimer's disease, and dementia," was published in *Journal of Alzheimer's Disease*.

Attention skinny people—you may get dementia. That's the finding from a study of more than two million people that looked at the relationship between body mass index (BMI) in middle age and dementia later in life. This study received a lot of press because it found, essentially, that the thinner you are, the greater your dementia risk…which goes against what most people might think and implies that there's no need to worry about staying trim.

Before you break out the cheesecake to celebrate, though, let's take a closer look.

"Contradicting Everything We Thought We Knew"

The researchers used a health-care database from a network of primary-care practices in the United Kingdom to find height/weight measurements on people aged 40 and older. They followed these people until they either left the network, were diagnosed with any form of dementia or died.

The result was more than a little surprising: Dementia risk decreased with each bump up in BMI. People who were underweight (BMI 20 or lower in this study, or under 139 pounds for a 5'10" tall person) had a 34% higher risk than average of developing dementia over 20 years than average—maybe not so surprising, since being underweight is obviously not a healthy thing to be. But then the higher that people went up on the weight spectrum, the lower their risk for dementia became, and that seemed downright odd. At the far end of the weight scale, those who were morbidly obese in midlife, with a BMI of 40 or higher (279 pounds for a 5'10" person) had a 29% lower risk for dementia than average. Crazy, huh?

Like all observational studies, the UK weight study has some inherent limitations. While these kinds of studies are valuable for pointing researchers toward associations, they can't show cause and effect. *Beyond this general limitation, there are specific concerns about this particular study's methods...*

Easy Way to Keep Alzheimer's Away

Walking six miles weekly may prevent Alzheimer's.

Recent finding: In a study of 426 adults with or without cognitive decline, those who walked at least six miles weekly were half as likely to develop Alzheimer's disease over 13 years as nonwalkers. Among those with cognitive impairment, walking five miles a week reduced cognitive decline by more than half.

Theory: Exercise improves blood flow to the brain, which helps keep neurons healthy.

To help preserve brain health: Aim to walk at least three-quarters of a mile daily.

Cyrus Raji, MD, PhD, physician-scientist, department of radiology, University of Pittsburgh.

•**It included mixed age groups.** You had to be 40 or older to be included, but there was no upper limit. Some people were 80 years old when their baseline info was recorded. (No matter how you slice it, being 80 isn't middle-aged.) So it's hard to draw conclusions from this data about how weight in middle age affects dementia risk when you're older. During midlife, a person normally gains weight. At around 65 or 70 years old, a person typically loses skeletal muscle and gains fat, but overall, BMI tends to decrease. Mixing up data from these two very different stages of life, means the study is not going to work.

•**It likely missed many cases of dementia.** Patients with dementia were identified only through a review of medical records in this study, but people may come into the health-care system with more acute illnesses that mask dementia, so this approach misses many late-onset cases of dementia. A better approach would be to conduct thorough evaluations among a representative sample, which can take hours, followed by discussion among more than one expert to confirm the diagnoses. It's expensive to conduct a study with time-consuming evaluations, which is why it can't be done on two million people. But it's more accurate.

•**It didn't distinguish between different types of dementia.** Certain hereditary forms of dementia tend to strike earlier in life. Early-onset dementia is a different beast, so it would have helped if the researchers had separated dementias diagnosed before age 65 from those diagnosed after age 65. Late-onset dementia may be influenced by being overweight, while early-onset dementia is more likely to be hereditary and influenced by specific genes.

What Do We Really Know About Weight and Dementia?

•**Watch your weight in midlife.** Studies investigating the association between midlife BMI and risk for dementia demonstrated generally an increased risk among overweight and obese adults. One reason may be that excess weight increases your risk for high blood pressure, high cholesterol levels and diabetes. All of these factors have been shown to increase the risk for dementia.

•**Being too skinny over the age of 70 increases your risk.** Being underweight (BMI 18.5 or lower) is associated with increased dementia risk. That's quite thin, such as 5' 4" and 107 pounds. No one is sure why, but there may be metabolic abnormalities that keep people underweight that also contribute to dementia risk. In some cases, the dementia process may begin decades before clinical symptoms and lead to a lower body weight.

•**A little extra weight in later life may be protective.** There is a consistent finding in the medical literature that over age 70, having a BMI in the "overweight" range (25 to 29.9) is protective. Some, but not all, studies find that even being obese (BMI 30 to 34.9) protects, too. If you're a little heavier going into late life, you may be less likely to develop dementia. While no one is sure why, it may be that fat tissue produces hormones that are protective for the brain.

It's not quite as much fun as a headline that says being fat is a good thing for your brain and memory. That would be nice for people who are heavy. But the real story appears to be that a healthy lifestyle that helps keep weight in the normal range throughout your middle years and into your 70s is good for your brain, too. Once you get into your 70s, a little extra weight may be fine.

At any age, however, a healthy diet and exercise is important for body—and mind. All of the things that we have been promoting for a long time—eating right and getting physical exercise—are actually relevant for dementia, too.

Loneliness Doubles Alzheimer's Risk

Robert S. Wilson, PhD, senior neuropsychologist of the Rush Alzheimer's Disease Center, Rush University Medical Center, Chicago.

For some time we've known that social isolation is a risk factor for dementia. A recent study goes far deeper, with findings offering fascinating insight. Researchers at Rush University in Chicago and the University of Pennsylvania followed 823 people older than 70 for four years, using questionnaires administered by researchers to assess social isolation and conducting tests of cognitive functioning. They discovered that people who scored highest on the loneliness scale—regardless of whether or not they actually spent much time with people—were more than twice as likely to develop AD during the follow-up period as people whose score was the lowest.

Who Gets Alzheimer's...and Who Doesn't

Loneliness is sometimes considered an early sign of AD, but these findings show it is associated with increased risk and not an early symptom of its pathology.

Culturally, we've been inclined to regard problems of age to be inevitable with the passing of years. This study shows it's time to correct that assumption and more closely investigate ways to prevent the debilitation of old-age diseases including dementia. The kind of loneliness this study talks about is more like a trait than an emotional state—it's not the type of loneliness you might experience being away from home for an extended period, which is loneliness as a state, but rather the type that you feel all or most of the time, loneliness as a trait, that follows you everywhere. Even so, there are still many ways to address and modify it. Medicine helps treat depression, which is usually part of loneliness, but non-drug therapies including regular exercise, joining like-minded groups for activities and expanding your circle of friends and acquaintances in general can be hugely beneficial—most especially when you've got strong networks already in place. If you live alone, you may want to consider moving to a retirement community, where even shy people can make connections, since most residents are looking to do so. Not only will being with others possibly help people avoid Alzheimer's in years to come, it will make for happier years right now.

Low Blood Pressure May Harm the Brain

Majon Muller, MD, PhD, geriatrician, VU University Medical Center Amsterdam, the Netherlands.

It's long been known that high blood pressure in middle age may cause brain shrinkage, or atrophy, later in life. But when 663 middle-aged patients with coronary artery disease or other vascular conditions were followed for about four years, those with low diastolic (bottom number) blood pressure readings (under 60 mm/Hg) also showed signs of atrophy.

Theory: Low blood pressure may be inadequate for healthy blood flow to the brain, which can lead to brain tissue loss. More research is needed to determine if low pressure should be treated to minimize risk for brain atrophy.

Hearing Loss Is Linked to Memory Loss

Study of 1,984 people, ages 75 to 84, by researchers at The Johns Hopkins University School of Medicine, Baltimore, published in *JAMA Internal Medicine.*

Older adults with even mild-to-moderate hearing loss may experience a decline in brain function up to 41% faster—or three years sooner—than those who have not become hearing impaired.

Reasons: When people are faced with hearing loss, the brain works harder to process sounds rather than dedicating energy to memory and thinking. And the social isolation that occurs among people with poor hearing may result in cognitive decline.

CHAPTER 2

Signs of Dementia and Alzheimer's

How to Avoid the Memory Glitches That Cause Panic

Aaron P. Nelson, PhD, chief of neuropsychology in the division of cognitive and behavioral neurology at Brigham and Women's Hospital and an assistant professor of psychology at Harvard Medical School, both in Boston. He is coauthor, with Susan Gilbert, of *The Harvard Medical School Guide to Achieving Optimal Memory*.

With all the media coverage of Alzheimer's disease and other forms of dementia, it's easy to imagine the worst every time you can't summon the name of a good friend or struggle to remember the details of a novel that you put down just a few days ago.

Reassuring: The minor memory hiccups that bedevil adults in middle age and beyond usually are due to normal changes in the brain and nervous system that affect concentration or the processing and storing of information. In fact, common memory "problems" typically are nothing more than memory errors. Forgetting is just one kind of error.

Important: Memory problems that are frequent or severe (such as forgetting how to drive home from work or how to operate a simple appliance in your home) could be a sign of Alzheimer's disease or some other form of dementia. Such memory lapses also can be due to treatable, but potentially serious, conditions, including depression, a nutritional deficiency or even sleep apnea. See your doctor if you have memory problems that interfere with daily life—or the frequency and/or severity seems to be increasing. *Five types of harmless memory errors that tend to get more common with age...*

31

MEMORY ERROR #1: Absentmindedness. How many times have you had to search for the car keys because you put them in an entirely unexpected place? Or gone to the grocery store to buy three items but come home with only two? This type of forgetfulness describes what happens when a new piece of information (where you put the keys or what to buy at the store) never even enters your memory because you weren't paying attention.

My advice: Since distraction is the main cause of absentmindedness, try to do just one thing at a time.

Otherwise, here's what can happen: You start to do something, and then something else grabs your attention—and you completely forget about the first thing.

We live in a world in which information routinely comes at us from all directions, so you'll want to develop your own systems for getting things done. There's no good reason to use brain space for superfluous or transitory information. Use lists, sticky notes, e-mail reminders, etc., for tasks, names of books you want to read, grocery lists, etc. There's truth to the Chinese proverb that says, "The palest ink is better than the best memory."

Helpful: Don't write a to-do list and put it aside. While just the act of writing down tasks can help you remember them, you should consult your list several times a day for it to be effective.

MEMORY ERROR #2: Blocking. When a word or the answer to a question is "on the tip of your tongue," you're blocking the information that you need. A similar situation happens when you accidentally call one of your children by the name of another. Some patients are convinced that temporarily "forgetting" an acquaintance's name means that they're developing Alzheimer's disease, but that's usually not true.

Blocking occurs when the information that you need is properly stored in memory, but another piece of information is getting in the way. Often, this second piece of information has similar qualities (names of children, closely related words, etc.) to the first. The similarity may cause the wrong brain area to activate and make it harder to access the information that you want.

My advice: Don't get frustrated when a word or name is on the tip of your tongue. Relax and think about something else. In about 50% of cases, the right answer will come to you within one minute.

MEMORY ERROR #3: Misattribution. This is what happens when you make a mistake in the source of a memory.

More than a few writers have been embarrassed when they wrote something that they thought was original but later learned that it was identical to something they had heard or read. You might tell a story to friends that you know is true because you read about it in the newspaper—except that you may have only heard people talking about it and misattributed the source.

Misattribution happens more frequently with age because older people have older memories. These memories are more likely to contain mistakes because they happened long ago and don't get recalled often.

My advice: Concentrate on details when you want to remember the source of information.

Focus on the five Ws: Who told you…what the content was…when it happened…where you were when you learned it…and why it's important. Asking these questions will help to strengthen the context of the information.

MEMORY ERROR #4: **Suggestibility.** Most individuals think of memory as a mental videotape—a recording of what took place. But what feels like memories to you could be things that never really happened. Memories can be affected or even created by the power of suggestion.

In a landmark study, researchers privately asked the relatives of participants to describe three childhood events that actually happened. They were also asked to provide plausible details about a fourth scenario (getting lost in a shopping mall) that could have happened, but didn't.

A few weeks later, the participants were given a written description of the four stories and asked to recall them in as much detail as possible. They weren't told that one of the stories was fictional.

What happened: About 20% of the participants believed that they really had been lost in a shopping mall. They "remembered" the event and provided details about what happened. This and other studies show that memories can be influenced—and even created—from thin air.

My advice: Keep an open mind if your memory of an event isn't the same as someone else's. It's unlikely that either of you will have perfect recall. Memories get modified over time by new information as well as by individual perspectives, personality traits, etc.

MEMORY ERROR #5: **Transience.** You watched a great movie but can't remember the lead actor two hours later. You earned an advanced degree in engineering, but now you can hardly remember the basic equations.

These are all examples of transience, the tendency of memories to fade over time. Short-term memory is highly susceptible to transience because information that you've just acquired hasn't been embedded in long-term storage, where memories can be more stable and enduring.

This is why you're more likely to forget the name of someone you just met than the details of a meaningful book that you read in college—although even long-term memories will fade if you do not recall them now and then.

My advice: You need to rehearse and revisit information in order to retain it. Repeating a name several times after you've met someone is a form of rehearsal. So is talking about a movie you just watched or jotting notes about an event in a diary.

Revisiting information simply means recalling and using it. Suppose that you wrote down your thoughts about an important conversation in your journal. You can review the notes a few weeks later to strengthen the memory and anchor it in your mind. The same technique will help you remember names, telephone numbers, etc.

Don't Panic If You Draw a Blank: Here's What's Dangerous

Majid Fotuhi, MD, PhD, neurologist, medical director of the NeuroGrow Brain Fitness Center in McLean, Virginia, and affiliate staff at Johns Hopkins Medicine, Baltimore. He is also author of *The Memory Cure* and coauthor of *The New York Times Crosswords to Keep Your Brain Young.*

Starting in their 40s, many people begin to have lapses in remembering names, occasional difficulty in finding a word and/or slowness in thinking speed (such as mentally adding numbers). Such occasional forgetfulness commonly occurs as we get older and is not necessarily a sign of dementia, as many people fear.

However, memory lapses that occur several times every day could be a sign of an underlying health problem and should be evaluated.

Many health conditions, including depression, thyroid problems and dehydration, can affect memory. Too much stress, too little sleep or a deficiency of vitamin B-12 can make someone forgetful, too.

Many medications, including tricyclic antidepressants, antihistamines and drugs that treat high blood pressure and cholesterol, can also cause memory loss. Your doctor may be able to prescribe other drugs that don't have this side effect.

Signs that memory lapses may be more serious include becoming lost in familiar places, asking the same question repeatedly and getting confused about time, people and places. If any of these signs occur, consult a neurologist.

Inability to Spot Lies May Warn of Dementia

Katherine P. Rankin, PhD, a neuropsychologist and associate professor of neurology at the University of California, San Francisco, Memory and Aging Center and coauthor of a study presented at a meeting of the American Academy of Neurology.

D oes someone you love seem increasingly gullible? Don't be too quick to dismiss this as a normal sign of aging. *Here's why...*

A recent study included 175 people ages 45 to 88, more than half of whom were in the early stages of some type of neurodegenerative disease that causes certain parts of the brain to deteriorate. Participants watched videos of two people talking. In addition to truthful statements, the video dialogue included sarcasm and lies, plus verbal and nonverbal clues to help participants pinpoint the false or insincere statements. Participants then answered yes/no questions about the video...and researchers compared their scores with results of MRI scans that measured the volume of different brain regions.

Results: Cognitively healthy people easily picked out the lies and sarcasm in the video, as did most participants with certain neurodegenerative diseases, including Alzheimer's. However, participants whose brain scans showed degeneration of the frontal and temporal lobes, a condition called frontotemporal dementia—which is as common as Alzheimer's disease among people under age 65—found it very difficult to distinguish factual statements from untruthful or sarcastic ones.

Bottom line: Increasing inability to recognize deception or sarcasm merits a consultation with a neurologist, especially if accompanied by other possible symptoms of frontotemporal dementia, such as severe changes in behavior and/or personality—yet often these are mistaken for signs of depression, a midlife crisis or normal aging. Early diagnosis of frontotemporal dementia may maximize treatment options and help protect patients vulnerable to being scammed due to their blind trust.

Worried That a Loved One Might Have Dementia? Questions to Ask

John C. Morris, MD, director, Charles F. and Joanne Knight Alzheimer's Disease Research Center, Washington University School of Medicine, St. Louis.

I t's an increasingly common problem—someone you care about seems to be showing signs of cognitive slippage, but you're not sure whether it's serious enough to merit testing or not. Should you schedule an appointment to see what the doctor thinks?

Not so fast. It turns out that the best person to judge whether or not there's a real reason to worry may not be a medical professional but a family member or close friend, a recent study shows. If this doesn't seem particularly surprising to you (after all, who better to evaluate changes in cognitive function than those who know a person best?), you may still find the study results startling—because a standard screening test used by health professionals to detect dementia was so much less effective in recognizing serious situations than the observations of family and friends.

Researchers at the Washington University School of Medicine in St. Louis wanted to see which of two tools to identify early-stage dementia worked better. One, called the Ascertain Dementia 8 (AD8) questionnaire, consists of an eight-question survey that is completed by a family member (usually the spouse or an adult child) or a friend of the person whose cognitive function is in question. The other is the commonly used Mini Mental State Exam (MMSE), a more detailed dementia screening test that is administered to the patient by a health-care professional. Researchers compared the results when both tests were used to evaluate 257 individuals (average age 75.4 years), some of whom were cognitively normal while others had mild Alzheimer's symptoms. Then they examined these people using imaging and spinal fluid tests that identify Alzheimer's changes in the brain, such as amyloid plaque. Although there were some "false positive" results, the AD8 questionnaire (the one done without using a doctor) picked up all but five of 101 individuals with dementia...while the MMSE test missed 74 of these mildly affected individuals!

Moreover, the AD8 is free, noninvasive and easy to complete in just a few minutes.

The AD8 questionnaire itself is not a diagnostic instrument but a reliably sensitive screening tool to determine the need to seek definitive diagnostic evaluation for Alzheimer's. Instead of just saying, "Dad's not really remembering to pay the bills like he used to," this questionnaire can give you a way to structure your concerns and then present them to your physician.

Here's the Test

To administer the questionnaire, answer the following yes-or-no questions regarding the loved one you're concerned about. Two or more "yes" answers may mean that further diagnostic testing is in order.

Over the last several years, have you noticed a change in cognitive abilities for your loved one in regard to...

- **Having problems with judgment** (e.g., problems making decisions, bad financial decisions, problems with thinking).

- **Showing less interest in hobbies/activities.**

- **Repeating the same things over and over** (questions, stories or statements).

- **Having trouble learning how to use a tool, appliance or gadget** (e.g., computer, microwave, remote control).

- **Forgetting the correct month or year.**

- **Having trouble handling financial affairs** (e.g., balancing a checkbook, income taxes, paying bills).

- **Having trouble remembering appointments.**

- **Having daily problems with thinking and/or memory.**

If you answered yes to two or more questions, don't panic—the AD8 isn't a diagnostic tool, but one that is meant to determine whether more testing should be done. To families facing uncertainty about what to do about a loved one who seems to be declining, this looks like a safe, wise and supportive first step to take.

The Nose Knows...

Sniff Test for Alzheimer's

A simple sniff test can help in the early diagnosis of Alzheimer's disease (AD).

Details: Researchers administered a test to identify 16 common odors to healthy patients and those diagnosed with mild cognitive impairment (MCI) or AD. Patients with MCI or AD scored lower than healthy patients. The sniff test combined with a standard cognitive test was 98% accurate at identifying patients who had AD, versus 93% for the cognitive test alone. If you're concerned about your memory, ask your doctor about getting the sniff test along with cognitive testing.

David R. Roalf, PhD, research assistant professor, department of psychiatry, University of Pennsylvania, Philadelphia.

Early Alzheimer's Sign?

Difficulty identifying certain smells, such as lemon or smoke, could signal Alzheimer's disease 10 years before the onset of memory loss, according to a new study of older adults.

Why: Alzheimer's can cause brain circuits to lose memory of certain smells.

Self-defense: If you or a loved one has difficulty identifying familiar smells, talk to your doctor about screening for Alzheimer's disease.

Mark Albers, MD, PhD, assistant professor of neurology, Harvard Medical School, Boston.

When Dementia Doesn't Start with Memory Loss

James M. Ellison, MD, MPH, the Swank Foundation Endowed Chair in Memory Care and Geriatrics at Christiana Care Health System in Wilmington, Delaware, and a professor of psychiatry and human behavior at the Sidney Kimmel Medical College of Thomas Jefferson University in Philadelphia.

Jane thinks she needs new eyeglasses because she's having trouble reading and seeing objects right in front of her. Joe's personality has dramatically changed, with the formerly genteel man making impulsive purchases and saying rude things. And Jack has begun to make things up, telling his family members grandiose stories they know aren't true.

What do all three have in common? You might never guess that each is suffering from dementia—a devastating condition that most people associate with memory loss.

It's true that declining thinking and reasoning skills, including memory loss, are signature characteristics of the "Big 3"—Alzheimer's disease, vascular dementia and Lewy body disease—which account for about 90% of all dementia cases.

However, the red flags suffered by the other 10% of dementia patients are surprising to many people because they deviate from "typical" symptoms, especially when the disease first develops. *Dementias that don't fit the norm...*

• **Posterior cortical atrophy (PCA).** Visual problems—such as blurry vision, difficulty reading and/or problems with depth perception and identifying objects—can signal PCA, which often strikes in one's mid-50s to early-60s. But these vision issues aren't caused by an eye condition. Instead, they stem from shrinkage in the back of the brain, where the occipital lobes, which control vision, are located.

PCA is actually a visual variant of Alzheimer's or frontotemporal dementia, with the brain no longer properly interpreting what the eyes are seeing. Other symptoms, including diminished memory, reasoning and other cognitive skills, can occur at the same time as the visual disturbances or can come on after a year or two.

How it's diagnosed: If a person is having vision issues, a visit to the eye doctor (an ophthalmologist or optometrist) can determine if he/she needs glasses or contacts or a new prescription. An eye doctor will also test for macular degeneration, cataracts and other eye problems.

If there are no issues with vision, the patient should see a neurologist, who can perform an exam and order imaging tests. When PCA is present, structural brain scans such as a CT or an MRI will likely show shrinkage in the brain's occipital lobes. These scans can also rule out other potential causes of symptoms, such as a stroke or tumor.

Treatment approaches: The same medications that may temporarily boost brain cell function in people with Alzheimer's can also help some people with PCA. These drugs include cholinesterase inhibitors, such as *donepezil* (Aricept), *rivastigmine* (Exelon) or *galantamine* (Razadyne), as well as *memantine* (Namenda), which blocks a particular brain receptor to enhance the effectiveness of synapses.

To make daily life easier and safer, PCA patients can ask a certified geriatric care manager (usually a social worker or nurse) to assess their homes. To find one in your area, contact the Aging Life Care Association at AgingLifeCare.org.

Examples of what helps: Removing clutter…labeling drawers and items… installing better lighting…and making glass doors and windows more visible with stickers.

•**Frontotemporal dementia (FTD).** Changes in personality, behavior, language or movement may point to FTD, which accounts for about 5% of all dementia cases. Often diagnosed between one's mid-40s and early-60s, FTD is caused by progressive nerve cell loss in the frontal lobes, an area in the front of the brain responsible for cognitive functions including problem solving, memory and judgment, and the temporal lobes, which are involved in short-term memory and emotion.

Uncharacteristic and even disruptive behavior changes are often the first noticeable symptoms of FTD, with patients becoming more irritable, impulsive, euphoric or compulsive. As the disease progresses, people with a language variant of FTD will eventually become mute or have more trouble speaking or understanding others. Memory loss is also a later feature of FTD.

How it's diagnosed: In addition to assessing clinical symptoms, a neurologist will use imaging tests such as CT or MRI scans, which may show wasting in the brain's frontal and temporal lobes, to help diagnose FTD. Additionally, about one-third of FTD cases are inherited, so genetic testing can be performed in those with a family history.

Treatment approaches: The medications most often used by Alzheimer's patients don't always ease FTD symptoms—and may actually worsen them. But other medications, including antipsychotics and antidepressants, can target specific symptoms as they arise. For example, some of the selective serotonin reuptake inhibitor (SSRI) antidepressants, such as *citalopram* (Celexa), may help behavioral symptoms, such as irritability.

Behavioral programs run by hospitals, dementia centers or psychologists can also help FTD patients and give their families the information they need to support their loved ones. Consult The Association for Frontotemporal Degeneration (TheAFTD.org) for information.

•**Korsakoff syndrome.** This disorder is triggered by a severe thiamine (vitamin B-1) deficiency, typically stemming from alcohol abuse or bariatric surgery. Because thiamine is needed to help brain cells convert glucose to energy, its absence causes brain damage that can lead to bizarre symptoms (see below).

Those with Korsakoff syndrome have a type of short-term memory loss (anterograde amnesia) that prevents them from learning new information and remembering recent events. Also, they may speak coherently and appear normal but "confabulate"—that is, they make up things they can't recall and may even believe their made-up stories.

How it's diagnosed: Since Korsakoff syndrome is typically preceded by a condition known as Wernicke encephalopathy—an acute, life-threatening brain reaction to lack of thiamine—it's easier to diagnose. Wernicke encephalopathy is characterized by impaired walking, confusion and abnormal eye movements. With the presence of these symptoms, a thiamine blood test can be used to support diagnosis.

Treatment approaches: Oral thiamine supplements will help about one-quarter of those with Korsakoff syndrome to recover (although it may take weeks or months). For others, thiamine deficiency causes permanent brain damage. These patients may need institutional care if their impairment is severe.

What a Good Physical Tells About Your Brain

Richard Carmona, MD, FACS, MPH, president of the Tucson, Arizona–based Canyon Ranch Institute and vice chairman of Canyon Ranch, a health resort, spa and wellness retreat. He served as US Surgeon General from 2002 to 2006 and is author of *Canyon Ranch 30 Days to a Better Brain.*

Put yourself on a weight-loss diet, and you can measure your success with a bathroom scale. If fitness is your goal, you can track your improvement by charting how fast you can run or walk a mile.

But how can you tell if your brain is as fit as the rest of you?

If you're having memory problems, that's an obvious red flag. But even if you're basically healthy (or are being treated for a chronic condition such as high blood pressure), a routine medical exam can tell a lot about your brain health—if you know what the seemingly basic tests may mean. *What a physical checkup reveals about your brain—and the additional tests you may need...*

Lay It All Out

Doctors aren't mind readers—they don't know what you're worried about unless you tell them. At your physical, tell your doctor about any changes in your health (even if you think they sound trivial).

Where most people get tripped up: There's always that routine question about medications you're taking. Don't assume that your doctor knows everything he/she has prescribed—include every medication and supplement you're taking.

Many common prescription or over-the-counter drugs—alone or in combination—can affect your brain. The following types of drugs are among the most commonly associated with dizziness, fuzzy thinking and/or memory problems. *All drugs within each class can addle a person's brain—not only the specific drug examples given...*

•**Allergy medications, including antihistamines** (such as Benadryl and Claritin).

•**Antianxiety medications** (such as Valium and Xanax).

•**Antibiotics** (such as Cipro and Levaquin).

•**Antidepressants** (such as Prozac and Lexapro).

•**Blood pressure medications** (such as Zestril and Procardia).

•**Sleep aids** (such as Ambien).

If you are taking one of these types of medications and are experiencing cognitive problems, ask your physician about switching to a different drug.

Fortunately, the fuzzy thinking and/or problems with memory usually go away when the drug is discontinued. And because everyone responds differently to individual medications, you may be able to safely take a different drug that's within the same class.

Clues from Your Physical

Even if you're not having cognitive problems, your physical can give you a measure of key markers of brain health. For example, most people know that high blood pressure is linked to increased risk for certain types of dementia (normal blood pressure is 120/80 or below). But low blood pressure (lower than 90/60) may make you dizzy, fatigued and unable to think clearly. *Other important brain-health markers…*

•**Eyes.** When your doctor shines that bright light in your eyes, he is looking at the retina, the light-sensitive tissue at the back of the eye that is connected directly to the optic nerve leading to the brain. Blood vessels in the retina reflect vascular health in the whole body—including the brain.

•**Hearing, balance and coordination.** While many diseases can cause problems with hearing, balance or coordination, one possibility is dysfunction of the eighth cranial nerve, which connects directly to the brain. Ears have fluid-filled canals that relay information to the brain via the eighth cranial nerve and act as a kind of gyroscope, giving us our sense of orientation in space. When we change position, the fluid moves, and the brain adjusts our balance and coordination. With some inner-ear disorders, such as Ménière's disease or labyrinthitis, people are dizzy, lose hearing or fall frequently due to loss of balance and coordination.

•**Reflexes.** A tap on your knee with a tiny hammer sends an electrical impulse to the spinal cord, which then sends a signal back to the foot, triggering a kick. A weak or delayed response could indicate a problem with the nervous system or brain.

•**Sensation.** All of the senses are housed in the brain, including the sense of touch. Any change in sensation—tingling hands or feet…weak hands…and/or numbness anywhere in the body—could signal a problem in the brain.

Digging Deeper

If your memory is failing or you're having other cognitive problems, such as difficulty making decisions or planning activities, your doctor may want to run tests for…

•**Inflammation.** A blood test for *C-reactive protein* (CRP) measures general levels of inflammation in the body. High levels of CRP (above 3.0 mg/L) could be due to a simple infection…cardiovascular disease that may also be putting your brain at risk…or an autoimmune disease, such as lupus or multiple sclerosis, which can cause problems with memory and thinking as well as physical symptoms.

•**Vitamin deficiencies.** A vitamin B-12 deficiency can lead to memory loss, fatigue and light-headedness. Other common nutrient deficiencies that can affect thinking include vitamin D and omega-3 fatty acids—there are tests for both.

•**Diabetes and glucose tolerance.** Left untreated, diabetes can dramatically increase one's risk for dementia. If your doctor suspects you have diabetes (or it runs in your family), get your blood glucose level tested (following an overnight fast).

Useful: An HbA1C test, which gives a broader picture of your glucose level over the previous six to 12 weeks. While most people, especially after age 45, should get glucose testing at least every three years, it's particularly important for those having cognitive symptoms.

•**Tick-borne illness.** Lyme disease and Rocky Mountain spotted fever can cause mental fuzziness.

Also helpful: Liver function tests, including new genomic tests, also may be ordered to assess your liver's ability to remove toxins. If the body doesn't clear toxins, this can alter brain metabolism, possibly leading to cognitive decline.

Questions to Ask If You Are Diagnosed with Alzheimer's Disease

Alzheimer's Association, American Academy of Neurologists, Harvard Medical School, Mayo Clinic.

A diagnosis of Alzheimer's can be terrifying. But the more you know about what to expect, the better off you'll be. *If your doctor tells you that you have Alzheimer's disease, here are important questions to ask...*

Are you sure it's Alzheimer's disease? Doctors can diagnose "probable Alzheimer's disease" with about 90% accuracy. But there's always room for error because many forms of dementia can mimic Alzheimer's. Ask your doctor how he/she will confirm that you actually have Alzheimer's and not another form of dementia that could possibly be more treatable (such as dementia caused by thyroid problems or a vitamin deficiency).

What will happen to me first? With early Alzheimer's, you might notice occasional (and slight) memory lapses. Your cognitive abilities will continue to worsen over time. Some people misplace things, and some make poor decisions or engage in uncharacteristically aggressive behavior. Your doctor can tell you what's typical for each of the three stages of Alzheimer's, but the specific symptoms will vary from person to person.

How will my moods change? You might become suspicious of close friends or family members. You might get angry more than you used to or become increasingly agitated toward the end of each day. If you do notice mood changes, ask your doctor what you can do to cope. In some Alzheimer's patients, certain behavior changes are due to something else altogether—such as depression.

What medications are you going to prescribe for me, and why? Depending on your symptoms and stage, you might be given *donepezil* (Aricept) or *memantine* (Namenda). A newer drug, Namzaric, combines both of these drugs in a one-a-day capsule. The drugs can help improve memory/confusion and delay the worsening of symptoms, although they cannot cure the disease. You might need other drugs—such as antianxiety medications—as well.

Could nondrug treatments make a difference in my case? Preliminary research finds that omega-3 fatty acids may slow cognitive declines in Alzheimer's patients who are missing a particular gene. (The US Food and Drug Administration recommends no more than three grams daily from food and supplement sources combined.) A supplement called huperzine A (a moss extract) has shown some benefit—it has properties that are similar to some Alzheimer's drugs. Check with your doctor before starting (or continuing to take) any supplement.

Should I increase my exercise? There's some evidence that vigorous exercise can slow or temporarily stop cognitive declines in those with an early stage of Alzheimer's disease. But hard exercise isn't safe for everyone—and it might or might not help. Your doctor can help you design the best exercise program for you.

Is it safe for me to drive? Personal safety is always an issue as Alzheimer's progresses. The American Academy of Neurologists says that no one with Alzheimer's (regardless of the stage) should drive a car, though other experts advise deciding case-by-case. Get your doctor's opinion on your situation.

CHAPTER 3

Alzheimer's Imposters

It Might Not Be Alzheimer's

Jacob Teitelbaum, MD, board-certified internist and founder of Practitioners Alliance Network. He is the primary investigator on a nationwide study using MIND to treat Alzheimer's and dementia and creator of the popular Cures A-Z app. Based in Kona, Hawaii, he is author, with Bill Gottlieb, of *Real Cause, Real Cure.*

If a doctor says that you or a loved one has Alzheimer's disease, take a deep breath and get a second opinion. Studies have shown that between 30% and 50% of people diagnosed with Alzheimer's turn out not to have it.

Bottom line: The symptoms common to Alzheimer's can be caused by other reversible conditions. Problems with memory and other cognitive functions often are linked to what I call MIND—metabolism, infection or inflammation, nutrition or drug side effects—or a combination of these factors. Addressing these can markedly improve cognitive function. Even people who do have Alzheimer's will see improvements.

Metabolism

Anyone who is experiencing confusion, memory loss or other cognitive problems should have tests that look at the hormones that affect metabolism. *In particular…*

• **Thyroid hormone.** A low level of thyroid hormone often causes confusion and memory loss. It also increases the risk for Alzheimer's disease. In recent studies, thyroid levels on the low side in the normal range are associated with a 240% higher risk for dementia in women. Borderline low thyroid hormone is associated with as much as an 800% higher risk in men.

My advice: For most people with unexplained chronic confusion and memory loss, I recommend a three-month trial of desiccated thyroid (30 mg to 60 mg) to see if it helps. It is a thyroid extract containing the two key thyroid hormones. (The commonly prescribed medication Synthroid has just one of the two.) If you have risk factors for heart disease—such as high LDL cholesterol and high blood pressure—your doctor should start you with a low dose and increase it gradually.

• **Testosterone.** This hormone normally declines by about 1% a year after the age of 30. But in one study, men who went on to develop Alzheimer's disease had about half as much testosterone in their bloodstreams as men who did not.

Every 50% increase in testosterone is associated with a 26% decrease in the risk for Alzheimer's.

My advice: Men should ask their doctors about using a testosterone cream if their testosterone tests low—or even if it's at the lower quarter of the normal range. Limit the dose to 25 mg to 50 mg/day. More than that has been linked to heart attack and stroke.

Infections and Inflammation

You naturally will get large amounts of protective anti-inflammatory chemical compounds just by eating a healthy diet and using supplements such as fish oil and curcumin. For extra protection, take aspirin. In addition to reducing inflammation, it's among the best ways to prevent blood clots and vascular dementia, which is as common as Alzheimer's disease. In addition, infections leave us feeling mentally foggy. Have your doctor look for and treat any bladder and sinus infections.

My advice: Talk to your doctor about taking one enteric-coated low-dose (81-mg) aspirin daily to improve circulation and reduce the risk for ministrokes in the brain. Even people with Alzheimer's may have had a series of ministrokes, adding to their cognitive decline. This is especially important when mental worsening occurs in small distinct steps instead of gradually.

Nutrition

The typical American diet is just as bad for your brain and memory as it is for your heart. Too much fat, sugar and processed food increase cell-damaging inflammation throughout the body, including in the brain.

In one study, Columbia University researchers studied more than 2,100 people over the age of 65 who consumed healthy foods such as nuts, fruits, fish, chicken and leafy, dark green vegetables and who limited their consumption of meat and dairy. They were 48% less likely to be diagnosed with Alzheimer's over a four-year period. *Especially important…*

•**B-12.** Millions of older adults don't get or absorb enough vitamin B-12, a nutrient that is critical for memory and other brain functions. You might be deficient even if you eat a healthful diet due to the age-related decline in stomach acid and intrinsic factor, a protein needed for B-12 absorption.

My advice: Take a multivitamin that contains 500 micrograms (mcg) of B-12 and at least 400 mcg of folic acid and 50 mg of the other B vitamins. If you test low-normal for B-12 (less than 400 ng/ml), also ask your doctor about getting a series of 10 B-12 shots.

Helpful: Have one teaspoon of apple cider vinegar with every meal. Use it in salad dressing, or mix it into eight ounces of vegetable juice or water. It will increase B-12 absorption.

Caution: Vinegar is highly caustic if you drink it straight.

•**Fish oil.** The American Heart Association advises everyone to eat fish at least twice a week. That's enough for the heart, but it won't provide all of the omega-3 fatty acids that you need for optimal brain health. Fish-oil supplements can ensure that you get enough.

My advice: I recommend three to four servings a week of fatty fish, such as salmon, tuna, herring or sardines. Or take 1,000 mg of fish oil daily. You will need more if you're already having memory/cognitive problems. Ask your doctor how much to take.

•**Curcumin.** Alzheimer's is 70% less common in India than in the US, possibly because of the large amounts of turmeric that are used in curries and other Indian dishes.

Curcumin, which gives turmeric its yellow color, reduces inflammation and improves blood flow to the brain. Animal studies show that it dissolves the amyloid plaques that are found in the brains of Alzheimer's patients.

My advice: Unless you live in India, you're not likely to get enough curcumin in your diet to help, because it is poorly absorbed. Use a special highly absorbed form of curcumin (such as BCM-95 found in CuraMed 750 mg), and take one to two capsules twice a day.

Caution: Taking curcumin with blood thinners can increase the risk for bleeding.

Alzheimer's Could Be This Dangerous Deficiency

Irwin Rosenberg, MD, senior scientist and former director, Nutrition and Neurocognition Laboratory, Tufts University, Boston.

It may seem like an extreme form of wishful thinking to suggest that symptoms believed to signal the onset of Alzheimer's disease could instead be due to a lack of one particular vitamin—and yet studies over the years have been telling us just that. Some people 50 and older who are suffering from memory problems, confusion, irritability, depression and/or paranoia could see those symptoms dramatically diminish simply by taking vitamin B-12.

Frighteningly, recent research shows that up to 30% of adults may be B-12 deficient—making them vulnerable to misdiagnosis of Alzheimer's. For years, doctors had believed that B-12 deficiency showed itself most significantly as the cause of anemia (pernicious anemia), but they now realize the lack of B-12 may even more dramatically be causing neurological symptoms, some of which are similar to Alzheimer's.

Others at Risk...

Age is not the only risk factor for having a B-12 deficiency—other at-risk groups include vegetarians (dietary B-12 comes predominantly from meat and dairy products) and people who have celiac disease, Crohn's disease or other nutrient malabsorption problems. Evidence accumulating over the past few decades shows that regular use of certain medications also can contribute to vitamin B-12 deficiency. These include antacids, in particular proton pump inhibitors (PPIs) such as *esomeprazole* (Nexium), *lansoprazole* (Prevacid) and many others which reduce stomach acid levels, making it difficult for B-12 to be fully absorbed. The diabetes drug *metformin* (Glucophage) also can reduce B-12 levels.

Measuring Deficiency

A common symptom of vitamin B-12 deficiency is neuropathy, a tingly and prickly sensation, sometimes felt in the hands and feet and occasionally in the arms and legs as well. People with B-12 deficiency also tend to have problems maintaining proper gait and balance. I recommend testing B-12 levels for a few groups of people, including those on PPIs for more than a few months...people having memory problems and/or often feeling confused—and this can include people of any age…those with neuropathy in the feet and/or legs…and those who have unexplained anemia.

As mentioned above, deficiencies of B-12 in older adults are nearly always a direct result of too little stomach acid, which is essential for absorption of B-12. This explains why powerful antacids trigger B-12 deficiency. Another problem is that sometimes, especially in older people, the stomach isn't making enough of a protein called *intrinsic factor* (IF) that is needed to break down B-12 effectively. There is no way to increase IF, and so the solution is to administer B-12 in large enough quantities to override the difficulty with absorption. Traditionally this has been done with injections of B-12, but more recently doctors have found that oral supplementation with high amounts of B-12 that dissolves under the tongue also is successful and certainly easier than regular injections. There is no reason to be concerned about "balancing" B vitamins as was once thought—B-12 is water soluble and the body can excrete what it doesn't need.

What You Can Do

Adults can easily get the recommended daily amount of 2.4 micrograms (mcg) of B-12 from dietary sources, which include all animal products. For example, just three ounces of steamed clams supplies 34.2 mcg and three ounces of salmon provides the necessary 2.4 mcg. However, this amount will not address the problems associated with aging and medications. Once again, the issue goes back to absorption—if you don't have enough stomach acid and/or IF to use the B-12 you ingest, it is almost irrelevant how much animal protein you eat. This is why the Institute of Medicine says that for people over age 50 and for vegetarians, the best way to ensure meeting your body's B-12 needs is to take a supplement or seek out foods fortified with it.

Reason: The body can more easily absorb the form of B-12 used for supplementation and fortification even in people who have low levels of stomach acid.

Caution: B-12 tests are sometimes insufficiently sensitive, especially for vegans. If your test indicates levels are fine in spite of symptoms, have your doctor order a different test that will evaluate whether your B-12 system is intact. There is no need to suffer from any kind of B-12 deficiency symptoms, let alone risk misdiagnosis of Alzheimer's, when the solution is so close at hand!

This Vascular Condition Causes Memory Loss...How to Stop It

Majid Fotuhi, MD, PhD, neurologist, medical director of the NeuroGrow Brain Fitness Center in McLean, Virginia, and affiliate staff at Johns Hopkins Medicine, Baltimore. He is also author of *The Memory Cure* and coauthor of *The New York Times Crosswords to Keep Your Brain Young.*

Alzheimer's disease is the most widely recognized form of dementia. But there's another cause of memory loss that people should know about—but usually don't.

Vascular cognitive impairment (VCI), which is typically caused by multiple small strokes, has been estimated to affect 1% to 4% of adults over age 65. However, because there is no agreement on the exact definition of this condition, the actual number of affected individuals is not known. Most older adults with vascular risk factors—such as high blood pressure (hypertension) and diabetes—may have varying levels of VCI.

Blood Vessels and Your Brain

The brain requires a hefty amount of blood—about 20% of the heart's output—to function normally. Even a slight reduction in circulation—such as that caused by small strokes—can result in symptoms, including slowed thinking, that can mimic Alzheimer's disease.

While genetics can play a role in Alzheimer's disease, VCI is widely recognized as the most preventable form of dementia. Even if you've begun to suffer early signs of this form of cognitive impairment (see symptoms on page 51), you may be able to avoid the devastating effects of full-blown dementia.

Hidden Blockages

Most people imagine stroke as a life-threatening event that causes dramatic symptoms. This is true of major strokes. It is not the case with ministrokes, also known as transient ischemic attacks (TIAs).

When Johns Hopkins researchers looked for evidence of microscopic strokes—areas of brain damage that are too small to be visible on a magnetic resonance imaging (MRI) scan—they found that such strokes are extremely common. Millions of Americans with normal cognition, including healthy adults, have probably experienced one or more of these minor ministrokes.

What happens: Small, transitory blood clots can momentarily prevent circulation to small areas of the brain. Or *vascular hypertrophy*, an abnormal growth of cells inside blood vessels, may impede normal circulation. In either case, certain parts of the brain receive insufficient blood and oxygen. The damaged areas can be much smaller than a grain of rice.

Symptoms—assuming that there are noticeable symptoms—tend to be minor. People who have experienced multiple ministrokes that affect larger or more diverse areas of the brain are those most likely to develop dementia, but it might take years or even decades before the problem is severe enough to be diagnosed. *Symptoms to watch for...*

•**Specific symptoms of VCI depend on the part of the brain affected.** Patients who have suffered multiple ministrokes may walk or think more slowly than they did before. Some have trouble following directions. Others may feel apathetic or confused.

•**Some ministrokes, however, affect only the part of the brain involved in decision-making and judgment.** The changes might be so subtle that a patient isn't aware of them—at least, until subsequent ministrokes affect larger or different areas of the brain.

Getting the Right Diagnosis

People who exhibit marked cognitive changes usually will be given an MRI or computed tomography (CT) scan. These tests sometimes reveal white, cloudy areas in the brain (infarcts) that have suffered damage from impaired circulation due to ministrokes.

Often, however, the ministrokes are too small to be detected. In these cases, patients may be incorrectly diagnosed with Alzheimer's disease. (The abnormal proteins that are characteristic of Alzheimer's cannot be detected by standard imaging tests.)

The distinction is important. There is no cure for Alzheimer's disease. In patients with VCI, there are a number of ways to stop the disease's progression and maintain long-term cognitive health.

Better Vascular Health

Brain damage that's caused by ministrokes can't be reversed. Medication—including cholinesterase inhibitors, such as *donepezil* (Aricept)—may modestly reduce some symptoms in patients with dementia but cannot cure it.

Preventive strategies, however, can be very effective in people with VCI alone. *Most important...*

•**Don't let high blood pressure shrink your brain.** Chronic hypertension is one of the main causes of dementia because the vascular trauma is constant. People with uncontrolled hypertension actually have smaller brains because of impaired circulation. Their risk of developing dementia is two to three times higher than that of people with normal blood pressure.

My advice: Blood pressure should be no higher than 120/80 mm Hg— and 115/75 mm Hg is better. Most people can achieve good blood pressure control with regular exercise and weight loss, and by limiting sodium and, when necessary, taking one or more blood pressure–lowering drugs, such as diuretics, beta-blockers or ACE inhibitors.

•**Avoid the other "D" word.** By itself, diabetes can double the risk for dementia. The actual risk tends to be higher because many people with diabetes are obese, which is also a dementia risk factor.

Important research: One study found that patients with multiple risk factors, including diabetes and obesity, were up to 16 times more likely to develop dementia than those without these risk factors.

My advice: By adopting strategies that prevent hypertension, including weight loss and regular exercise, you'll also help stabilize your blood sugar— important for preventing or controlling the health complications associated with diabetes.

•**Keep an eye on your waist.** Obesity increases the risk for hypertension and diabetes and has been associated with damage to the hippocampus (the brain's main memory center). Obese patients also have a much higher risk for obstructive sleep apnea, interruptions in breathing during sleep that can increase brain shrinkage (atrophy) by up to 18%.

My advice: Measure your waist. For optimal health, the size of your waist should be no more than half of your height. Someone who's 68 inches tall, for example, should have a waist measurement of 34 inches or less.

•**If you drink, keep it light.** People who drink in moderation (no more than two drinks daily for men or one for women) tend to have higher HDL, so-called "good," cholesterol...less risk for blood clots...and a lower risk for stroke and dementia.

My advice: If you already drink alcohol, be sure that you don't exceed the amounts described above. Drinking too much alcohol increases brain atrophy.

•**Get the right cholesterol-lowering drug.** People with high cholesterol are more likely to develop *atherosclerosis* (fatty buildup in the arteries) and suffer a ministroke or stroke than those with normal cholesterol levels.

My advice: Talk to your doctor about statins, such as *atorvastatin* (Lipitor) and *simvastatin* (Zocor). These drugs not only reduce cholesterol but also may fight blood-vessel inflammation. Other cholesterol-lowering drugs—such as resins, which bind in the intestines with bile acids that contain cholesterol and are then eliminated in the stool—don't provide this dual benefit.

Alzheimer's Could Be Depression... or a Stroke

Zaldy S. Tan, MD, MPH, medical director, Alzheimer's and Dementia Care Program, and associate professor, David Geffen School of Medicine, University of California, Los Angeles. He is author of *Age-Proof Your Mind: Detect, Delay and Prevent Memory Loss—Before It's Too Late.*

A lzheimer's disease is a devastating condition for which there is no effective treatment.

What you may not know: Certain people who think they have Alzheimer's actually may have a condition that is treatable. Unless the misdiagnosis is identified, these people will not only be given ineffective and potentially dangerous treatment, but their real problem also will go untreated. *Conditions that can mimic Alzheimer's...*

Depression

Cognitive impairments due to depression are known as *pseudodementia*. Because of a depression-induced lack of attention, which makes it difficult to form and process effective memories, patients may forget appointments or have difficulty remembering names. They also may have trouble concentrating, learning new things and even recognizing faces. This type of dementia, unlike Alzheimer's, is potentially reversible.

Distinguishing signs: Sleep disturbances are more likely to occur with depression than with early-stage Alzheimer's disease. For example, depressed patients may have early morning awakenings or experience difficulty falling asleep at night (typically marked by tossing and turning in bed). They can also have unexplained tearfulness as well as a lack of interest in things that they used to enjoy, a condition called *anhedonia.*

Treatment: If depression is the culprit, consider talk therapy or an antidepressant, such as *citalopram* (Celexa) or *sertraline* (Zoloft). An antidepressant can usually treat the forgetfulness associated with depression, but it may take several weeks to determine whether a particular drug/dose is going to work. You might also ask your doctor about Saint-John's-wort and other over-the-counter (OTC) natural remedies.

NPH

It's estimated that up to 200,000 older adults in the US have excessive accumulation of fluid on the brain, a condition known as *normal pressure hydrocephalus* (NPH). The fluid presses on the brain and can cause memory loss and other symptoms that may mimic Alzheimer's.

Distinguishing signs: Most patients with NPH have three main symptoms—an unsteady gait (in the early stages)…followed by urinary incontinence…and cognitive impairments (in later stages). With Alzheimer's, the order is reversed—memory loss and/or other cognitive problems occur first, followed in later stages of the disease by problems with bladder control and gait.

Treatment: NPH can potentially be corrected by inserting a shunt, a tube in the brain that drains excess fluid. However, the surgical procedure is not recommended until after the diagnosis is confirmed by an MRI of the brain and a trial removal of a small amount of fluid through a lumbar tap results in improved memory and/or gait. (For more information, see page 65 "This Alzheimer's Imposter is Treatable.")

Stroke

When a person has a series of ministrokes (warning strokes), it can lead to a type of vascular dementia known as multi-infarct dementia, which can be mistaken for Alzheimer's.

Multi-infarct dementia occurs when damaged blood vessels in the brain slow (but don't completely stop) normal circulation. Reductions in blood and the oxygen it carries can damage brain cells and impair memory and other cognitive abilities—but usually without the motor deficits that accompany a stroke, such as weakness of a limb or slow and/or garbled speech.

Distinguishing signs: Multi-infarct dementia can cause rapid changes in mental functions, sometimes within a few weeks to a month. With Alzheimer's disease, these changes typically occur slowly but steadily over several years.

Treatment: Multi-infarct dementia usually can be diagnosed with a CT or MRI scan showing characteristic changes in the brain. Unfortunately, existing brain damage can't be reversed, although future damage may be avoided. The goal of treatment is to prevent additional vascular damage and cognitive declines by treating the underlying risk factors, such as high blood pressure.

Stengler's Medical Mystery: Surprising Cause of Memory Loss

Mark A. Stengler, NMD, a naturopathic doctor and founder of the Stengler Center for Integrative Medicine in Encinitas, California. He is author or coauthor of numerous books, including *The Natural Physician's Healing Therapies* and *Bottom Line's Prescription for Natural Cures,* and author of the newsletter *Health Revelations.* MarkStengler.com

Memory lapses—as in, what is her name?—are an uncomfortable but generally inevitable part of the aging process. Sometimes these lapses are amusing—but there's only anxiety and fear, no humor at all, when memory decline creeps into and interferes with everyday life. This is what had begun to happen to 69-year-old Brad, a financial consultant whose professional success had brought him the home and lifestyle that a high-level career affords. Rather suddenly, Brad began to have trouble remembering things he'd just been told. He sometimes got lost while driving in areas he'd long known well. As a way to compensate he began to carry a pen and notepad at all times, constantly jotting down reminders about things people told him and tasks and errands he needed to do.

Different Doctors, Different Answers

Always an active and forceful person, Brad wasn't the type to simply accept that dementia might be setting in. Because his cholesterol levels were moderately elevated and he worried about his heart, the physician he saw most regularly was a cardiologist. When he called her to discuss his increasingly frequent memory lapses, she referred him to a neurologist for an evaluation. This doctor examined Brad, ran standard tests and gave him the much-feared diagnosis—it appeared he was in early-stage dementia, perhaps from vascular

How to Avoid "Statin Brain"

Statins can cause memory loss in some patients, despite a recent study that found they don't have cognitive side effects. The study was a generalized statistical study—not a personalized look at vulnerable patients. Some people who are susceptible do have "statin brain." Symptoms stop when the drug is stopped. These patients should talk to their doctors. Anyone considering starting a statin should ask about every-other-day rather than daily dosing.

Linda L. Restifo, MD, PhD, professor in the department of neurology at University of Arizona, Tucson.

problems or possibly as the first symptoms of Alzheimer's disease.

Facing this dire diagnosis prompted Brad to call me in the hope that a physician trained and experienced in treating illness with natural substances might offer a way to strengthen his memory and perhaps even ward off dementia. I first reviewed Brad's medical history, including when his memory problems started and how rapidly they had progressed. I quickly realized that this disturbing symptom first presented itself just a few months after Brad's cardiologist had put him on a statin drug (Lipitor) to lower his cholesterol. Knowing that statins have been anecdotally linked to a wide variety of side effects, including false dementia, I decided to investigate if a more natural protocol to lower Brad's cholesterol could replace the drug. Stopping the Lipitor without endangering Brad's cardiovascular health would determine if his dementia was real or a side effect of the drug. His cardiologist was informed of the treatment plan.

Natural Treatment Begins

This wasn't going to be merely a matter of substituting a vitamin regimen for his prescription drug, however. The first step prescribed was a diet to reduce Brad's LDL cholesterol (low-density lipoprotein, the potentially dangerous one). *It included...*

•**Regular consumption of soluble fiber,** including foods such as beans, barley, oats, peas, apples, oranges and pears. Soluble fiber reduces the absorption of cholesterol from the intestines into the bloodstream.

•**At least two servings a week (optimally four or more) of fish such as anchovies,** Atlantic herring, sardines, tilapia and ocean or canned salmon, specifically for their omega-3 fatty acids. This could also be accomplished with supplements.

•**A daily handful of nuts rich in monounsaturated fatty acids,** such as almonds and walnuts. A Spanish study found that a walnut-rich diet reduced total cholesterol by as much as 7.4% and LDL cholesterol by as much as 10%.

•**Ground flaxseeds**—up to a quarter-cup daily with 10 ounces of water or tossed into a salad or shake. This has been shown to reduce total and LDL cholesterol.

To manage his cholesterol, I also had Brad double his number of weekly aerobic exercise sessions, from twice each week to at least four times. I prescribed plant sterols, shown to reduce LDL cholesterol by up to 14%, recommending Beta sitosterol, which works by inhibiting cholesterol absorption in the digestive tract by up to 50%, without disrupting the more beneficial HDL cholesterol. I prescribed a 1.5 gram soft gel capsule to be taken with breakfast and dinner for a total of three grams daily. Brad would need to continue this regimen for life, since in taking his medical history I had learned that his elevated cholesterol had genetic roots.

Just Remember This...Many Meds Cause False Dementia

Once Brad went off Lipitor and onto his new program, his memory improved significantly. He has no need for memory-enhancing supplements, although he does take a multivitamin daily per my advice. I also monitor Brad's cholesterol levels regularly. They have remained in a normal range and Brad had no reason to return to statins.

Clearly Brad's memory problems were not symptoms of early dementia... but rather side effects of the statin drug. But statins are not the only drugs that may trigger side effects that mimic dementia. Other drugs that can cause these problems include tricyclic antidepressants and certain medications for Parkinson's disease—which is ironic in that PD itself can eventually cause dementia. Pain medications (narcotics such as *OxyContin* and *Vicodin*) can also cause memory problems, as can regular use of over-the-counter antihistamines including Benadryl, Chlor-Trimeton and Tavist.

These drugs have a common denominator: They all have anti-cholinergic properties, which means they suppress neurotransmitters that regulate certain aspects of mental functioning, especially those that relate to memory. This explains why anti-cholinergics can actually cause cognitive problems, and why the principal drugs to treat AD are in the pro-cholinergic category.

When concerned about memory lapses, many people today turn to a variety of supplements. A more effective strategy would be to schedule a visit to a naturopathic physician to review the medications they take regularly, both pharmaceutical and OTC, as these may be where the problem lies. In fact, a study published in the *British Medical Journal* reported on 372 elderly people without dementia who were taking anti-cholinergic medication. After following this group for eight years, the researchers found that 85% of this group had mild cognitive impairment, compared with 35% of the people in a second group who had never used the drugs. This is an important reminder why people and their doctors should wonder whether symptoms of early dementia might relate to medication—and therefore be reversible. That's advice worth remembering.

When "Dementia" Is Really Lyme Disease

Richard I. Horowitz, MD, an internist and medical director of the Hudson Valley Healing Arts Center in Hyde Park, New York. He has treated more than 12,000 patients with chronic Lyme disease over the past 30 years. He is a past president of the International Lyme and Associated Diseases Educational Foundation, and the author of *How Can I Get Better: An Action Plan for Treating Resistant Lyme & Chronic Disease.* CanGetBetter.com

People who have been told that they have Alzheimer's disease or another form of dementia owe it to themselves to ask their doctors one important question—"Could it be Lyme disease?"

Case in point: Singer Kris Kristofferson struggled for years with memory problems. His doctors suspected Alzheimer's disease or brain damage from sports-related head injuries.

He got some surprising news: What he really had was Lyme disease, which often causes cognitive problems that can be misdiagnosed as Alzheimer's disease.

What most people don't realize: While doctors routinely look for the physical symptoms of Lyme disease, such as a rash, fatigue, joint and muscle pain and unexplained fevers, many don't realize that psychological and cognitive impairments, including depression, anxiety, short- and long-term memory loss and other symptoms often confused with Alzheimer's disease, are also important clues.

The Brain at Risk

Lyme disease is a bacterial infection transmitted by tick bites. The organisms that can cause human infection readily travel from the place where a tick bite occurred into the brain, the sac surrounding the brain (the meninges) or the spinal cord as well as to the muscles, joints, heart and other parts of the body.

What happens next: Infection and inflammation of brain tissue can lead to memory and concentration problems and may also cause psychiatric problems, such as visual and auditory hallucinations that resemble schizophrenia. Infection of nerves in the spinal cord can cause numbness, tingling, burning or stabbing sensations in the arms and legs and/or across the trunk, which can come and go and even migrate to other parts of the body.

Shocking fact: About a quarter of all people diagnosed and treated early for Lyme disease go on to develop a chronic and hard-to-treat infection that often leads to some of the neurological symptoms described earlier, as well as headaches, neck stiffness, light and sound sensitivity and sleep disorders. The percentage is much higher among Lyme patients who aren't given early antibiotic treatment, who are undertreated or who remain undiagnosed.

Why It's Missed

Doctors should suspect Lyme disease when patients complain about problems with memory, concentration or other cognitive functions—particularly in parts of the country where Lyme and other tick-borne diseases are rampant (mainly the Northeast and upper Midwest). But Lyme is spreading. Doctors should consider it in dementia work-ups.

Experts advise Americans who live in tick-infested areas to be alert for the earliest sign of Lyme infection—a bull's-eye–shaped rash surrounding the site of the tick bite. However, only about 50% of Lyme patients ever develop a rash...or they confuse the rash with a spider bite, skin infection or bruise. Unless they know for a fact that they were bitten by a tick—and most don't— they don't even consider that Lyme might be the culprit.

More worrisome are the cognitive/psychological symptoms that affect more than 90% of the Lyme patients I've treated. These include memory loss and concentration problems, depression and psychiatric disorders...as well as symptoms easily mistaken for those caused by Alzheimer's disease and other neurodegenerative disorders.

Diagnostic complication: Even when Lyme is suspected, it's often difficult to diagnose. That's why doctors should start with a clinical diagnosis that is supported by lab testing. Hallmarks of Lyme include pain that migrates around the body and symptoms that come and go. When used together, the two main blood tests for Lyme disease—the Western blot and the ELISA test—miss about half of all infected patients. To improve accuracy, newer tests such as the C6 ELISA and EliSpot, which show higher sensitivity in detecting evidence of Lyme disease, can also be done. Other options (such as DNA and RNA tests, Nanotrap, etc.) are available, and spinal taps and PET scans may also be helpful.

Best advice: When outdoors, wear protective clothing treated with *permethrin* (an insect repellent), use tick sprays (those containing *IR3535* and *picaridin* are safer) and do frequent tick checks. Remove any ticks immediately using fine-tipped tweezers and grasping the tick as close to the skin as possible, pulling upward without squeezing. Save the tick so it can be tested and examined by your health-care provider.

Suspect Lyme disease if you experience *sudden* concentration or memory problems, anxiety and mood swings, headaches, migratory joint or muscle pain, dizziness or other symptoms—especially if you have no history of these problems. Such symptoms can occur within days to months of the bite.

Treatment Challenges

People who aren't treated quickly for Lyme (or those who have Lyme disease along with another tick-borne disease, such as *babesiosis* or *bartonellosis*) might not improve when they're given the standard antibiotic therapy—usually oral *doxycycline* (Oracea), *amoxicillin* (Moxatag) or *cefuroxime* (Zinacef). Because Lyme is more curable when treated early, your doctor might begin medication if you have symptoms (such as migratory joint pain) even before test results are confirmed or if you've had a tick bite but are not displaying symptoms of illness. About three-quarters of Lyme patients who take antibiotics within a month of the infection won't develop long-term symptoms and can be cured.

Important: If you've had antibiotic treatment for Lyme but continue to have neurological symptoms, the infection has likely spread to the nervous system. This may require different combinations of antibiotics for a longer treatment period. There are many treatment options, depending on specific symptoms, your medical history, the type of infection(s) and other considerations, such as allergies and the state of your immune and gastrointestinal systems.

How I have treated Lyme patients with persistent neurological symptoms: During the first month of treatment, I might prescribe *doxycycline* with *hydroxychloroquine* (Plaquenil), an antimalarial drug that helps to increase effectiveness, with or without the antibiotics *metronidazole* (Flagyl) or *tinidazole* (Tindamax) to kill cystic (dormant) forms of bacteria. I find that two or three drug regimens work best for chronically ill patients.

Important: Treatment must be tailored to the individual.

Anti-inflammatory Support

The presence of cognitive/psychological symptoms with Lyme disease always means that inflammation is affecting the brain and/or surrounding tissue. When you're infected, microglial cells in the brain secrete inflammatory substances that cause fatigue, mood changes and problems with memory and concentration. It's critical to shut down the infection and accompanying inflammation. *What helps…**

•**Anti-inflammatory supplements, such as curcumin, broccoli seed extract, resveratrol and green tea extract.** Take them one at a time or all together. Also consider an antioxidant such as glutathione.

•**Stevia, available in supplement form (the Nutramedix brand is effective), has been shown to kill the Lyme bacterium,** and it reduces and breaks up Lyme biofilms, "sheets" of bacteria that resist the effects of antibiotics. Gradually work up to 15 drops, twice a day. (*Note:* This is not the same stevia found in the sweetener section of the grocery store.)

•**A good night's sleep is critical during Lyme treatments.** Sleep deprivation increases inflammation…impairs immunity…and increases cognitive/ psychological symptoms.

•**An anti-inflammatory diet,** including lots of healthy, low-carbohydrate fruits and vegetables…no sugar…and little or no red meat. I often recommend a mercury-free fish oil supplement as well.

*If you use prescription medication, have a chronic medical condition or are pregnant or nursing, consult your doctor before taking any supplements.

Surprising Causes of Paranoia

Leslie Kernisan, MD, MPH, clinical instructor, division of geriatrics, University of California, San Francisco. Dr. Kernisan is board-certified in both geriatrics and internal medicine and founder of BetterHealthWhileAging.net, a website that provides practical information for older adults and family caregivers.

Your aging mother thinks her trusted caretaker is stealing money from her wallet. Your spouse suddenly believes he hears the voice of his grandson (who lives in another state) warning him that he's in imminent danger and telling him that he must leave the house immediately.

It can be frightening when a loved one experiences suspicious thoughts that have no rational basis—that is, paranoia. It's a common phenomenon, but it is not a normal sign of healthy aging. And contrary to what many people believe, it's not always dementia.

When the Brain Breaks Down

Paranoia involves intense or fearful feelings and thoughts related to persecution, threat or conspiracy. It's often, but not always, accompanied by delusions—believing something to be true that is false.

Acting paranoid is a sign that something is off-kilter with the brain. While we don't have reliable statistics for the causes of paranoia per se, my research has shown that we do have such data for the broader category of psychosis, a disconnect from reality, which is a reasonable stand-in because it often brings on paranoia.

At first glance, you might think psychosis is caused by schizophrenia. But that is the cause only 1% of the time. About 40% of the time, it's due to dementia, whether caused by Alzheimer's disease, Lewy body dementia or vascular disease.

What about the other 60%? There are many surprising causes—often eminently treatable. *Here are the main ones, described below in order of how quickly they can be addressed…*

An Underlying Condition

About 10% of the time, psychosis is caused by a physical illness, nutritional deficiency or other health condition unrelated to dementia, such as…

•**An imbalance of electrolytes**—crucial nutrients that help regulate heart rhythm and muscle function—including sodium, potassium, calcium and magnesium. It can be caused by chronic conditions such as kidney disease but also by a bout of flu that leads to vomiting and diarrhea.

•**Low levels of vitamins B-12 or folate—** both conditions are common in the elderly.

•**Infections, including pneumonia and urinary tract infections, which can be serious in the elderly.** Serious infections can cause delirium, a state of worse-than-usual mental function that can bring on paranoia.

•**A parathyroid tumor.** The parathyroid glands, located on the thyroid gland in the neck, can develop noncancerous tumors. These can stimulate the release of excess calcium into the bloodstream, which affects behavior and can lead to paranoia. It's curable with surgery.

> **Look Out for Changes in Speech Pattern**
>
> Changes in speech patterns may be an early sign of dementia.
>
> *Recent finding:* Aspects of language are affected much earlier than previously believed.
>
> *Example:* People who start to include more pauses and filler words, such as "um" and "uh," in their speech eventually could develop cognitive difficulties, such as Alzheimer's disease. Treatment of dementia-causing diseases typically is most effective when started early.
>
> Sterling Johnson, PhD, is a professor of psychology, University of Wisconsin-Madison.

These health problems can easily overwhelm an older adult. Once the underlying illness or deficiency is treated, however, the paranoia usually improves in a few days or, at most, weeks.

Important: The elderly experience thirst less intensely than younger people, often leading to dehydration. In individuals who already have mild memory problems, this can trigger a mild form of delirium, which often includes paranoia. Fortunately, reversal can be quick—give the person a glass of water or juice, and he/she will show signs of improvement in about 15 minutes.

Use Caution with These Medications

Certain drugs, as well as alcohol, can cause paranoia, especially in the elderly. These are responsible for about 10% of psychosis/paranoia cases. *Medications that are of particular concern…*

•**Benzodiazepines.** Drugs including *lorazepam* (Ativan), *diazepam* (Valium) and *alprazolam* (Xanax) are often prescribed to help people sleep or manage anxiety but can lead to paranoia.

Note: Stopping these drugs suddenly can be dangerous. Work with your doctor to discontinue them slowly.

●**Anticholinergics.** These drugs block the neurotransmitter acetylcholine—opposite to the mechanism of some Alzheimer's drugs, which make acetylcholine more available to the brain.

Chronic use—daily for two years or more—is linked with an elevated chance of developing dementia, and it's common for paranoia to be among the first symptoms that emerge. They are found in over-the-counter sleeping aids...drugs for overactive bladder, including *oxybutynin* (Ditropan) and *tolterodine* (Detrol)...and sedating allergy drugs such as *diphenhydramine* (Benadryl).

The Danger of Hospital Delirium

Delirium is responsible for approximately 10% of psychosis/paranoia cases. A common trigger is a hospital stay, especially one that includes surgery.

Rather than a single cause, delirium is often brought on by the rapid-fire combination of many destabilizing factors in a hospital stay—including over-medication (especially with painkillers, sedatives and sleeping pills), infection, isolation, dehydration, poor nutrition and sleep disturbance. Inadequately treated pain or constipation can also contribute to delirium.

Stunningly, experts estimate that about one-third of hospital delirium cases can be prevented. If your family member is slated for surgery, consult with a geriatric specialist at the hospital.

Very important: Ask if the hospital has an Acute Care for the Elderly (ACE) Unit, where specific measures are taken to keep geriatric patients mobile, well-rested, hydrated, out of pain and in regular contact with others.

Also helpful: Visit often and bring reminders of home such as family photos to ease feelings of isolation and disorientation.

Depression and Bipolar Disorder

Depression and bipolar disorder can bring on paranoid delusions, including the feeling of being punished. These conditions may be responsible for more than 30% of psychosis/paranoia in the elderly. Fortunately, effective treatment of the underlying disorders can reduce or eliminate the paranoia.

How to Get Help for Paranoia

If your loved one shows signs of paranoia, it's a safety issue, a health issue and a family crisis.

Do not attempt to reason with the person or explain why his/her paranoid thoughts are wrong. Instead, try to help the person feel heard and validated, then redirect if possible. If the person looks sick or unwell, is out of control or seems to be posing a serious risk of harming himself or someone else, consider the emergency room or even 911.

Next, insist on a thorough evaluation. Be persistent, because many doctors will just conclude that the person has dementia and leave it at that. This is especially important if paranoia symptoms come up suddenly—call the doctor for an urgent care appointment that includes evaluation for a new illness or medication side effect.

This Alzheimer's Imposter Is Treatable

Michael A. Williams, MD, director of adult and transitional hydrocephalus and CSF disorders at University of Washington Medical Center and professor of neurology and neurological surgery at University of Washington School of Medicine, both in Seattle. He is a past president of the International Society for Hydrocephalus and CSF Disorders and a founding member of the Adult Hydrocephalus Clinical Research Network. Dr. Williams is currently a member of the board of directors and medical advisory board of the Hydrocephalus Association.

If you're over age 65, it's common to feel that you're slowing down a bit. Simply walking to your mailbox could take longer than it used to, and you may have even started shuffling as you walk. Getting out of a chair could be getting harder, too.

On top of that, your bladder might not be cooperating, so you have started to wear pads for incontinence. Your thinking isn't quite as clear as it used to be, and you are now having trouble keeping your checkbook.

Don't make this mistake: While these changes all may seem to point to the fact that you're simply growing older, having all three of these symptoms could actually be a red flag for a treatable brain disorder.

As many as 700,000 people in the US are believed to have idiopathic (with no known cause) normal pressure hydrocephalus (iNPH), an often-misdiagnosed brain condition. Of the 5.2 million individuals diagnosed with dementia, estimates show that 10% to 15% actually have this treatable condition.

When It's Not Normal Aging

A shuffling gait, incontinence and memory problems may prompt a person to see his/her doctor, but these symptoms are also among the most common in older adults. For that reason, your doctor may chalk up these problems to "normal aging"—when, in fact, they are not normal.

If the patient is savvy and doesn't accept that answer, he/she will find another doctor and get a more extensive workup.

The turning point comes when the doctor orders a CT scan or an MRI—a test usually included in a dementia evaluation. If the imaging test shows that the brain's ventricles—normal cavities within the brain that contain cerebrospinal fluid (CSF)—are enlarged, that should trigger consideration of iNPH.

What's gone wrong: Hydrocephalus results from a defect in circulation of the CSF, which surrounds and cushions the brain. Normally, the *choroid plexus* (vascular tissue in the ventricles) produces up to 2.5 cups of CSF daily, which bathes the brain and is absorbed back into circulation, maintaining a constant volume of fluid inside the skull. If absorption slows down, then CSF accumulates, the ventricles enlarge and eventually symptoms (such as those described earlier) may appear.

Getting Diagnosed

If the brain scan shows enlarged ventricles, indicating possible iNPH, the next step is to see a neurologist for a clinical exam. The first symptom a neurologist will probably look for is a gait disturbance, including difficulty getting in or out of a seat, trouble initiating gait, shuffling gait and instability on turns. The presence of a shuffling gait along with cognitive slowing and memory impairment and/or urinary incontinence raises the diagnosis to "probable iNPH."

Important: Because cognitive defects caused by iNPH are frequently mistaken for Alzheimer's disease, a neurologist is best qualified to distinguish between the two types of memory loss.

Unlike Alzheimer's, iNPH usually does not reach the stage where the individual fails to recognize family or close friends. In addition, those with early Alzheimer's rarely display the distinctive gait impairment characteristic of iNPH, such as difficulty standing or turning, as mentioned above.

Unlike arthritis, the gait disturbance caused by iNPH is due to a neurologic impairment rather than pain or stiffness. Normal walking should be effortless, but individuals with iNPH must concentrate to walk and often complain that their feet won't do what they want them to do.

The slowness and shuffling of iNPH may cause it to be mistaken for Parkinson's disease, but the tremor that is typical of Parkinson's is not a key feature of iNPH. Patients with iNPH may even be prescribed medications for Alzheimer's, Parkinson's or incontinence, but these rarely help.

Another disorder that iNPH may resemble is vascular dementia, which is caused by the cumulative effects of various risk factors, such as high blood pressure, a history of small strokes, elevated cholesterol and diabetes. Because vascular dementia and iNPH often affect the same areas of the brain, the conditions can produce similar symptoms and sometimes even occur at the same time.

Getting the Right Treatment

It's important for iNPH to be treated. While there are no drugs for iNPH, the good news is that most cases can be treated by surgically implanting a shunt. The shunt consists of three components—a narrow tube that is placed in the ventricles…a valve mechanism to control the flow, which is usually placed beneath the scalp…and a narrow tube that transports excess CSF somewhere else in the body, usually to the abdominal cavity, where it's easily absorbed into the bloodstream.

To determine whether shunt surgery will help, tests of the patient's response to CSF removal are recommended. A spinal tap (also known as lumbar puncture) may be performed on an outpatient basis. With this procedure, approximately 30 milliliters (ml) to 40 ml, or nearly 1.5 ounces, will be removed. The patient's gait should be evaluated before the lumbar puncture and several hours afterward. If the gait improves significantly, then a shunt is very likely to help the patient.

If there's no improvement after the spinal tap, a more extensive test called external lumbar drainage (ELD) may be performed in the hospital. In this case, the doctor will insert a temporary tube into the spinal fluid to drain it for about four days, for an approximate total of 400 ml to 600 ml, or 13.5 ounces to 20 ounces, of CSF.

ELD is like a test-drive of shunt-like conditions for the brain, without actually having the shunt operation. If the patient shows improvement following prolonged drainage, he will then be referred for shunt surgery. If the patient does not respond to prolonged drainage, then the odds of a shunt helping are small—below 5%.

iNPH Care Lasts a Lifetime

Following shunt surgery, recovery rates for iNPH patients range from 60% to 90%, according to the medical literature. All symptoms can improve, but the extent of improvement may be limited if patients have other disorders that contribute to their symptoms.

It's important for people with shunts to visit the neurologist or neurosurgeon regularly following shunt surgery, initially to find the optimal setting for the shunt valve that controls drainage and on an ongoing basis to ensure that it's still operating correctly.

Too much drainage can increase the risk of bleeding within the skull, known as a subdural hematoma, and can cause symptoms such as headaches and nausea. Sometimes, therapy is useful to help patients regain balance and cognitive function.

Finding the Best Doctor

To find a neurologist or neurosurgeon who has experience diagnosing and treating iNPH, consult the website of the Hydrocephalus Association, which provides a directory of neurologists and neurosurgeons throughout the US, HydroAssoc.org/physicians-directories.

Stay Sharp as You Age—Surprising Causes of Memory Loss

Pamela W. Smith, MD, MPH, codirector of the master's program in metabolic and nutritional medicine at Morsani College of Medicine at University of South Florida and owner/director of the Michigan-based Center for Personalized Medicine. She is author of *What You Must Know About Memory Loss & How You Can Stop It: A Guide to Proven Techniques and Supplements to Maintain, Strengthen, or Regain Memory.* CFHLL.com

It is no secret that age and memory are intertwined. But age itself is not the sole reason that we forget things. Memory loss often can be traced to specific factors, including hormonal changes, inflammation and exposure to mercury and other toxins.

Common causes of memory loss—and what you can do to control them...

Impaired Circulation

If you have high cholesterol or other cardiovascular risk factors—you smoke, have high blood pressure, are sedentary, overweight, etc.—you probably have at least some atherosclerosis, fatty plaques in the arteries that reduce the flow of blood and oxygen to the brain.

What to do: In addition to the obvious—more exercise, weight loss, not smoking—I strongly advise patients to eat a Mediterranean-style diet. This features lots of fruits, vegetables and grains along with healthy amounts of olive oil and fish. A recent study found that people who closely followed this diet were 28% less likely to develop mild cognitive impairment and 48% less likely to get Alzheimer's disease.

Also helpful: Eating more soluble fiber (such as that found in oatmeal, beans, fruit and nuts) or taking a fiber supplement has been shown in both men and women to decrease hardening of the arteries and improve circulation.

Exposure to Mercury

Americans are exposed to mercury all the time. It is present in soil, the water supply and some foods, including many fish. It also is used in many dental fillings. Over time, the mercury from fillings and other sources can cause inflammation and oxidative stress in the brain, both of which can damage the neurotransmitters that are essential for memory and other brain functions.

What to do: You can get tested for mercury and other heavy metals, but the tests will be positive only after long-term exposure. I advise patients to reduce their exposure long before it will show up on any test.

If you have dental fillings made of amalgam (an alloy of mercury and other metals), consider replacing them with fillings made from plastics or other materials. The work should be done by an environmental dentist who specializes in the safe removal of mercury.

Also important: Avoid eating shark, swordfish, king mackerel, marlin, orange roughy, ahi tuna and tilefish, which tend to accumulate mercury. Limit canned albacore tuna to three servings or less per month and canned light tuna to six servings or less per month.

Best: Cold-water salmon.

Your Drugs May Give You Dementia

Sam Gandy, MD, PhD, professor of neurology and psychiatry at the Mount Sinai School of Medicine in New York City.

A diagnosis of dementia could be your worst nightmare, but what may be even more troublesome is the possibility of being told you have dementia, when in fact one simple step could reverse it quite simply. "Pseudodementia" is far more common than you'd guess…and the cause can often be found in your medicine cabinet.

I see many elderly patients who seem to be suffering from Alzheimer's disease (AD) or other forms of dementia…but may not be. As many as 10% of those 65 and older believed to have dementia may actually be experiencing side effects from medication.

Sleeping pills are a common culprit. A good night's sleep often becomes increasingly elusive for aging men and women, leading doctors, sympathetic to their plight, to prescribe drugs such as *zolpidem* (Ambien). These drugs trigger mental and physical lethargy—that's why they work—but in some people that state of mind and body carries over to the next day and impairs function. It's not just prescriptions, either—over-the-counter sleep-aids, which seem as innocent as popping a vitamin, can also cause this problem. OTC sleep-aids (including brands like Unisom SleepTabs, Tylenol PM and Nytol QuickCaps caplets) contain antihistamines, virtually all of which can cause dementia-like symptoms.

Yet another common type of drug prescribed to elderly patients to promote sleep and/or calm nerves are tranquilizers in the benzodiazepine class. This includes *lorazepam* (Ativan), *clonazepam* (Klonopin), *alprazolam* (Xanax), diazepam (Valium) and many more. Occasional use is okay, but when people take such medications often, they can build up in the system, leading to dementia-type symptoms. If you are going to take a "benzo," look for one with a short half-life such as Ativan or Xanax rather than, say, Valium, which lingers much longer in the body, thus making accumulation more likely.

Beyond Sleeping Pills—What Else?

Still other drugs used to treat frequent medical problems in the elderly can slow cognition. These include some beta blocker drugs, prescribed for a wide variety of problems such as high blood pressure, irregular heart rhythm, migraine, angina and glaucoma. Also, anticholinergic drugs are a problem—these are prescribed to treat Parkinson's disease, chronic obstructive pulmonary disease (COPD), some gastrointestinal problems, urine retention and more. Although some studies seem to have shown that statin drugs (the world's top-selling pharmaceuticals, prescribed to lower cholesterol levels) help prevent dementia, there is considerable anecdotal evidence of people developing dementia symptoms after taking them—with symptoms then vanishing when they stop the drug. Drugs are often lifesavers, but not all that much is known about what happens in the body when they are used over long periods, and most especially in combination with other medications. This is one of the most important reasons why it is smart to take as few medications as possible.

Yet another frequent cause of pseudodementia is not a drug, but rather depression—a condition that is particularly complicated in the elderly because they tend to isolate themselves and often their depression symptoms closely resemble early-stage dementia. In fact, I've had experiences of trying to set up a clinical trial for Alzheimer's disease, only to discover that candidates referred by their physicians actually suffered clinical depression, not AD at all. Treating these patients with antidepressants also improved their cognition.

What You Can Do

The resounding message is that no one should be quick to accept a diagnosis of dementia as the cause of memory loss and/or confusion, especially in an elderly individual. Call your doctor if you develop memory problems soon after starting a new drug. Have your doctor scrutinize all medications to see if one or the combination might be causing the symptoms. Be sure your pharmacist has a complete list of all medications taken, especially if they aren't all filled at the same pharmacy. If it turns out that one or several of the drugs you take could be the cause, work out a plan with your doctor to withdraw from the drug or drugs for a month or so to see if symptoms change. Finally, be very careful about any sleep aids, whether OTC or prescription.

Over-the-Counter Drug-Induced Memory Loss

Malaz Boustani, MD, MPH, associate director, Indiana University Center for Aging Research, Indianapolis.

D rug-induced memory loss may occur after just 60 days of antihistamine use. These anticholinergic drugs are in a class of medication that also includes many blood thinners, antidepressants and medications used for overactive bladder, heart disease and chronic obstructive pulmonary disease.

In a recent study of 3,690 adults, those who took a daily dose of a strong anticholinergic drug, such as *diphenhydramine* (Benadryl), for 60 days had mild cognitive impairment, including memory loss.

If you regularly take an anticholinergic: Talk to your doctor about switching to a different drug. *Cetirizine* (Zyrtec) has far fewer anticholinergic side effects and can be used for allergies.

Foggy and Forgetful? The Problem Could Lie in the Liver

Lisa M. Forman, MD, is an associate professor of medicine in the division of gastroenterology and hepatology and the director of the Gastroenterology Fellowship Program at the University of Colorado School of Medicine in Aurora. Her research interests include hepatic encephalopathy, hepatitis C, liver transplantation and metabolic complications after liver transplantation. Dr. Forman is a member of the Alpha Omega Alpha Honor Medical Society.

A woman started making so many mistakes at work that despite her decade of supercompetent service to the company, she was in danger of being fired. Noting her mom's growing confusion, concentration problems and uncharacteristic irritability, her daughter wondered if Alzheimer's was setting in. But then the mother's doctor diagnosed a completely different problem called hepatic encephalopathy (HE), a brain disorder that develops when the liver is unable to remove toxic substances from the blood. Toxins such as ammonia then build up and travel through the bloodstream to the brain, impairing cognitive function.

HE most often develops in people with cirrhosis (scarring of the liver) caused by hepatitis C, alcoholism or other conditions. (The women above had contracted hepatitis many years before her concentration problems surfaced.) HE also can occur in the absence of cirrhosis in people who, for any of various reasons, develop acute liver failure. HE hospitalizes, on average, 200,000 individuals each year in the US. The condition can be acute or chronic.

Symptoms of HE can worsen gradually or suddenly. Mild HE symptoms include poor concentration, forgetfulness, mild confusion, mood problems, impaired math and handwriting skills, changes in sleep patterns and a musty, sweet odor to the breath. More severe symptoms include lethargy, apathy, disorientation, slurred speech, obvious personality changes, marked confusion and amnesia. In very severe cases, HE patients may experience brain swelling, then lapse into a coma and die.

Diagnosing the problem: The early symptoms of HE can be subtle, so it's easy for doctors to miss them. At a checkup, the patient might seem completely coherent—aware of the date and who the current president is, for instance. But then a family member will point out that the patient's driving reflexes are slow, almost as if she were driving while intoxicated, or that the patient is having trouble focusing, or that she sometimes stays awake at night and sleeps during the day. Another possible clue that can appear in the early or later stages is a phenomenon called asterixis, in which (for reasons that are not fully understood) the hands flap uncontrollably when the arms are extended.

While various tests can provide useful information, there is no laboratory or imaging test that can definitively diagnose HE. Thus, the diagnosis depends on excluding other possible causes for a patient's dementia-like symptoms, given that various conditions can mimic HE... and, in cases in which a liver problem had not been previously detected, identifying the underlying disorder.

Help for HE: In some cases of acute HE, the condition can be reversed by addressing the underlying cause of the liver dysfunction. For chronic HE, treatment centers on minimizing symptoms. *Treatment options may include...*

•**Avoidance of factors and/or prompt treatment of conditions that could increase the buildup of toxins in the bloodstream**—for instance, constipation, dehydration, electrolyte disturbances, kidney problems, infection or the use of medications that tax the liver.

•**Dietary changes that help reduce formation of ammonia and other toxins and/or speed the passage of food through the intestines.** For instance, patients may be instructed to limit animal protein and increase fiber consumption.

•**Medication.** Because the toxins responsible for HE arise from the gut, a laxative drug called lactulose may be used to speed the passage of food through the digestive tract and to help bind toxins so they can be eliminated in the stool. Antibiotics also may be prescribed to inhibit ammonia-producing bacteria in the gut.

Exciting development: The FDA has approved the antibiotic *rifaximin* (Xifaxan) for treating HE. Rifaximin has been proven to decrease repeat HE episodes as well as hospitalizations and, unlike other antibiotics prescribed for HE, it has no serious negative side effects.

•**HE can lead to rapid deterioration**—so if the above measures are not enough to keep the condition under control, a liver transplant may be the best option. In that case, a patient should be referred to a transplant center to begin the evaluation process. For many transplant patients, receiving a new liver cures the HE.

CHAPTER 4

Help for Cancer and Other Brain Dangers

How a Top Brain Doc Protects His Own Brain from Cancer

Keith Black, MD, chairman of the department of neurosurgery and director of Maxine Dunitz Neurosurgical Institute at Cedars-Sinai Medical Center, Los Angeles. He is author, with Arnold Mann, of *Brain Surgeon: A Doctor's Inspiring Encounters with Mortality and Miracles.*

A large study that examined data over a 20-year period found that the incidence of brain tumors had increased by 200% in older adults. In children age 14 years and younger, primary brain tumors are now the most common cause of cancer. But is brain cancer really on the rise—or simply more likely to be detected? *A noted expert discusses the research and what he does to protect his own brain...*

Is the Increase Real?

CT scans are an important tool for diagnosing brain tumors. Before they were introduced in the 1970s, many patients with tumors might have been misdiagnosed as having strokes or other neurological diseases. The increased use of CT scans—along with MRIs and brain biopsies—may have caused an apparent increase in brain tumors.

Using research that took into account better imaging technology, scientists at the National Brain Tumor Registry concluded that the incidence of new tumors has remained stable. The National Cancer Institute Brain Tumor Study found a slight decrease in the incidence of brain tumors between 1990 and 2002.

However, the data is murky. There does appear to be an increase in brain tumors in some populations, but it still is unclear if this is due to better diagnostic tests or other factors (such as extended cell-phone use).

We know that secondary brain tumors (those that originate in other parts of the body) are about five times more common than primary tumors (ones that originate in the brain and tend to stay in the brain)—in part, because many people with cancer now are living long enough for the cancer to spread to the brain.

About 30% of those who die from breast cancer are later found to have evidence of brain cancer. With lung cancer, about 60% will be found at autopsy to have had the cancer spread to the brain.

Reduce the Risk

Primary brain cancers are relatively rare, accounting for about 2% of all cancers. It is estimated that 26,000 malignant cases will be diagnosed in 2018. Sadly, only about one-third of patients with brain or other nervous system cancers survive more than five years.

Brain tumors are difficult to treat. Surgery isn't always possible or effective, because these tumors tend to grow rapidly and invade large areas of brain tissue. Unlike other blood vessels in the body, those in the brain are selective in what they allow to pass. This so-called blood-brain barrier makes it difficult to deliver chemotherapeutic drugs to brain tumors.

The causes of brain cancer are largely unknown, but there are some clear risk factors...

•**Dental X-rays.** Most dentists routinely use X-rays during checkups.

The danger: Radiation scatters and can potentially irradiate—and damage—brain cells. Even low-dose X-rays may increase the risk for gliomas (a type of brain tumor) and meningiomas (tumors that develop in the membranes that cover the brain and spinal cord).

I tell my dentist, flat-out, that I don't want X-rays. An occasional X-ray probably isn't harmful, but no one should get them routinely.

•**Air pollution.** During a recent study we looked at the association between air pollution and brain cancers. Molecular changes in the brains of rats occurred after three months of exposure to air pollution that were similar to the changes we see just prior to the development of brain cancer.

•**Electromagnetic radiation from cell phones, cellular antennas and the like.** A Swedish study found that the risk for brain cancer is 250% higher in those who used a cell phone for up to an hour a day for 10 years.

This is controversial. Other, shorter-term studies have found no risk from cell-phone use. But we know that it typically takes 20 to 30 years before toxic exposures lead to cancer. Cell phones haven't been around long enough to know what the long-term consequences might be. (See page 80 for more studies on cell phones and brain cancer.)

My advice: Use a wireless earpiece when talking on a cell phone. If you don't use an earpiece, hold the phone as far away from your head as possible. The amount of radiation that reaches the brain drops significantly with distance.

Caution: Children have thinner skulls than adults. It's easier for electromagnetic radiation from cell phones to penetrate a child's skull and reach the brain. It's possible that even low levels of electromagnetic radiation can produce cancer-causing changes in brain cells. Children and young adults should always use an earpiece.

•**Hot dogs and other processed meats usually contain nitrites, substances that have been linked with brain tumors.** I like a hot dog as much as anyone, but moderation is important. Also, whenever possible, buy nitrite-free hot dogs, bacon and other processed meats.

•**Heating plastic in the microwave.** There isn't direct evidence that using plastic containers in the microwave can increase brain tumors, but we know that the vinyl chloride in some plastics is a risk factor. Personally, I don't use plastic containers or cover foods with plastic wrap in the microwave.

Pregnant women should be especially careful. We've found in animal studies that adult females exposed to vinyl chloride or other carcinogens might not develop brain tumors themselves, but their offspring face a much higher risk.

Four Supplements That Can Impair Your Brain

Cynthia Kuhn, PhD, professor of pharmacology, cancer biology, psychiatry and behavioral sciences at Duke University School of Medicine in Durham, North Carolina. Dr. Kuhn is also coauthor of *Buzzed: The Straight Facts About the Most Used and Abused Drugs from Alcohol to Ecstasy.*

I t is hardly news that supplements—just like drugs—can often cause physical side effects and reactions with prescribed medicines.

Recent development: Researchers are now learning more and more about unwanted mental changes that can occur when taking popular supplements (such as herbs and hormones).

These supplements can be a hidden cause of depression, anxiety, mania and other mental changes because patients—and their doctors—often don't realize how these products can affect the brain.

Supplements that may cause unwanted mental changes...

Melatonin

Melatonin is among the most popular supplements for treating insomnia, jet lag and other sleep disorders. Melatonin is a natural hormone that's released by the pineal gland at night and readily enters the brain. Unlike many sleep aids, it doesn't render you unconscious or put you to sleep—it causes subtle brain changes that make you "ready" for sleep.

Studies have shown that people who take melatonin in the late afternoon or early evening tend to fall asleep more quickly when they go to bed. The amount of melatonin used in scientific studies ranges from 0.1 mg to 0.5 mg. However, the products in health-food stores typically contain much higher doses—usually 1 mg to 5 mg. Supplemental melatonin also may become less effective over time, which encourages people to increase the doses even more.

Effects on the brain: In people with depression, melatonin may improve sleep, but it may worsen their depression symptoms, according to the National Institutes of Health.

What to do: Melatonin can help when used short term for such problems as jet lag. It is not particularly effective as a long-term solution for other causes of insomnia.

St. John's Wort

St. John's wort is probably the most studied herb for treating depression. Researchers who analyzed data from 29 international studies recently concluded that St. John's wort was as effective as prescription antidepressants for treating minor to moderate depression.

St. John's wort appears to be safe, particularly when it's used under the supervision of a physician. However, it can cause unwanted mental changes.

Effects on the brain: St. John's wort may increase brain levels of "feel good" neurotransmitters, including serotonin and dopamine. But unwanted mental changes that may occur in anyone taking St. John's wort include anxiety, irritability and vivid dreams. It may also lead to mania (a condition characterized by periods of overactivity, excessive excitement and lack of inhibitions)—especially in individuals who are also using antipsychotic drugs.

Caution: This supplement should never be combined with a prescription selective serotonin reuptake inhibitor (SSRI) antidepressant, such as *sertraline* (Zoloft) or *paroxetine* (Paxil). Taking St. John's wort with an SSRI can cause serotonin syndrome, excessive brain levels of serotonin that can increase body temperature, heart rate and blood pressure—conditions that are all potentially fatal. It also can interact with certain drugs such as oral contraceptives and immunosuppressant medications.

What to do: If you have depression, do not self-medicate with St. John's wort. Always talk to your doctor first if you are interested in trying this supplement.

Testosterone

Older men whose testosterone levels are declining (as is normal with aging) are often tempted to get a prescription for supplemental "T," which is advertised (but not proven) to improve their ability to get erections. Some women also use testosterone patches or gels (in much lower doses than men) to increase sexual desire and arousal.

Effects on the brain: If your testosterone is low, taking supplemental doses may cause a pleasant—but slight—increase in energy. However, with very high doses, such as those taken by bodybuilders, side effects may include aggression and mood swings. Men and women may experience withdrawal symptoms—such as depression and loss of appetite—when they stop taking it.

Testosterone replacement for men is FDA approved only for those with a clinical deficiency—defined as blood levels under 300 nanograms per deciliter (ng/dL).

What to do: Testosterone has been shown to increase sexual desire in women—it is not FDA approved for women but may be prescribed "off-label." The evidence supporting testosterone's ability to improve sexual function and well-being in normally aging men is weaker—unless they have been proven on more than one occasion to have low testosterone and related symptoms. Both men and women should take testosterone only under the supervision of a doctor.

Weight-Loss Supplements

Two ingredients that are commonly used in weight-loss supplements, beta-phenylethylamine (PEA) and P-synephrine, are said to increase energy and metabolism and burn extra calories.

Effects on the brain: Both PEA and P-synephrine (a compound found in supplements made from bitter orange) can make you feel jittery and anxious, particularly when they are combined with stimulants such as caffeine.

Many weight-loss and "energy" products are complicated cocktails of active ingredients that haven't been adequately studied—nor have they been approved by the FDA. They're risky because they've been linked to dangerous increases in blood pressure.

Important: There is little evidence that any of these products is particularly effective as a weight-loss aid.

What to do: Don't rely on weight-loss supplements. To lose weight, you need to decrease your food intake and increase your exercise levels—no supplement can accomplish that!

Can Your Cell Phone Cause Cancer?

Devra Davis, PhD, MPH, president of Environmental Health Trust, a nonprofit scientific and policy think tank focusing on cell-phone radiation. She is author of *Disconnect: The Truth About Cell Phone Radiation.* EHTrust.org

You may have heard that cell phones have been linked to cancer but wondered if that could really be true. A recent study offers strong evidence that this is the case—cell phones and other wireless devices emit a type of microwave radiation termed *radiofrequency radiation* (RFR) that can cause brain cancer and other cancers.

Here are the findings and what to do to minimize this risk to your health...

Recent Evidence

The government's National Toxicology Program (NTP) conducts scientific studies on toxins to see how they might affect the health of Americans. More than 90 studies show that the radiation emitted by cell phones and other wireless devices can damage DNA, the first step on the road to cancer.

In May 2016, the NTP published preliminary results from a two-year animal study on the health effects of cell-phone radiation—this was the largest study on animals and cell-phone radiation ever published.

One out of every 12 of the animals studied were affected by the radiation. Some of those that were exposed to daily, frequent doses of cell-phone radiation from birth developed *glioma,* a rare, aggressive type of brain cancer already linked to cell-phone use in people. (Glial cells surround and support neurons.) Other animals had precancerous changes in glial cells. And some developed rare tumors of the nerves around and within the heart called *schwannomas*. In contrast, a control group of animals not exposed to wireless radiation had no gliomas, no precancerous changes in glial cells and no schwannomas.

There are two crucial takeaways from this recent study…

1. For decades, many scientists and governments have embraced the following scientific dogma—the only unsafe radiation is "thermal" radiation that heats tissue, such as an X-ray. "Nonthermal" RFR doesn't heat tissue and therefore is safe. One study—during which animals exposed to RFR were monitored to ensure that there was no heating of tissue—contradicts this dogma.

2. Epidemiological studies that analyze health data from hundreds of thousands of people have linked gliomas and schwannomas to long-term cell-phone use—and this specific study found the same type of cancers in animals exposed to wireless radiation, strengthening the link.

Even More Dangers

Gliomas and schwannomas aren't the only dangers. *Research links wireless-device use to a range of other cancers, diseases and conditions…*

•**Meningioma.** A recent study published in *Oncology Reports* showed that heavy users of mobile and cordless phones had up to twice the risk for meningioma, cancer in the protective coverings that surround the brain.

•**Salivary gland (parotid) tumors.** Salivary glands are below the ear and in the jaw—exactly where many people hold cell phones during conversation. A study published in *American Journal of Epidemiology* showed a 58% higher risk for these (usually) noncancerous tumors among cell-phone users.

•**Acoustic neuroma.** Studies show that heavy or longtime users of cell phones have nearly triple the risk of developing acoustic neuromas (also called vestibular schwannomas), noncancerous tumors on the nerve that connects the inner ear to the brain. Symptoms can include gradual hearing loss and tinnitus in the affected ear, along with balance problems, headaches and facial numbness and tingling.

•**Breast cancer.** A study published in *Case Reports in Medicine* describes four young American women, ages 21 to 39, who had tucked their smartphones into their bras for up to 10 hours a day for several years. Each of them developed breast tumors directly under the antennas of their phones. None of the women had the cancer-causing BRAC1 or BRAC2 gene, a family history of cancer or any other known risk factors.

•**Male infertility and potency.** Several studies link close contact with wireless devices—wearing a cell phone on the hip or using a laptop computer on the lap—with fewer sperm, sluggish sperm, abnormally shaped sperm, sperm with damaged DNA and erectile dysfunction.

•**Sleeping problems.** Research shows that people who use cell phones and other wireless devices in the hours before bedtime have more trouble falling asleep and staying asleep. Both wireless radiation and the "blue light" from screens suppress melatonin, a sleep-inducing hormone.

How to Protect Yourself

Every step you take to reduce radiation is protective because exposure to radiation is cumulative—the higher the exposure, the higher your risk for cancer and other health problems.

The devices you should be concerned about include cell phones, cordless phone handsets and bases, Wi-Fi routers, wireless computers, laptops, iPads and other tablets, smartwatches, wireless fitness bands, iPods that connect to the Internet, wireless speakers, cordless baby monitors, wireless game consoles and any other type of wireless device or equipment such as thermostats, security networks, sound systems and smart meters.

•**Keep it at a distance.** To decrease your exposure to wireless radiation, keep wireless devices as far away from you as possible. *Just a few inches can make a big difference…*

•Never put the phone next to your head. Instead, use the speakerphone function or a wired headset or an earpiece.

•Never place a turned-on device in a pocket or jacket or tucked into clothing. Keep it in a carrier bag, such as a briefcase or purse. Never rest a wireless device on your body. This includes laptops and tablets—keep them off your lap.

•Never fall asleep with your cell phone or wireless tablet in the bed or under your pillow. Many people fall asleep streaming radiation into their bodies.

•**Prefer texting to calling.** And avoid using your cell phone when the signal is weak—radiation is higher.

•**Turn it off.** Putting your cell phone in "airplane" mode stops radiation. Also, look for the function key on your wireless device that turns off the Wi-Fi. Turn it off when the device isn't in use. There's also a function key to turn off

Bluetooth transmissions. If you must use a Wi-Fi router at home, locate it as far away from your body as possible. And turn it off at night.

To stop a gaming console from emitting radiation, you need to turn it off and unplug it.

•**Don't use your cell phone in metal surroundings such as a bus, train, airplane or elevator.** Using the phone creates radiation "hot spots" that increase exposure.

Exception: It is OK to use a cell phone in a car if your phone is hooked into the car's Bluetooth system—this reduces radiation to the user.

•**Trade in the cordless phone.** Cordless phones and wireless routers that use a technology called DECT emit as much radiation as cell phones whether you are using them or not. At home, install telephones that get their signal by being plugged into a jack. Forward your cell phone to your landline whenever you're home.

Dr. Mark Hyman's "UltraMind" Strategy for Brain and Mental Health

Mark Hyman, MD, author of *The UltraMind Solution: Fix Your Broken Brain by Healing Your Body First, UltraMetabolism* and *The UltraSimple Diet.* Dr. Hyman is founder and medical director of The UltraWellness Center in Lenox, Massachusetts. DrHyman.com

Mental illness is on the rise, and conventional medicine cannot cure it. An epidemic of "broken brains" affects millions of people worldwide, taking many forms—anxiety, depression, dementia, addictions, attention deficit hyperactivity disorder (ADHD), autism, etc. The common model for addressing these disorders is drug therapy…but drugs alone fail to address the underlying causes of mental disease.

The Shortcomings of Drug Therapy

The real cure for brain disorders lies outside the brain. If you suffer from depression, for example, you are not suffering from a "Prozac deficiency" in spite of the fact that doctors may prescribe it or other antidepressants. Mainstream medicine's approach is to make a diagnosis based on symptoms, then suppress those symptoms with a medication rather than identifying the cause and fixing that. For example, many cases of depression are actually rooted in nutritional deficiencies or imbalances, including vitamin D, B-12, an omega-3 fatty acid deficiency, or a problem with digestive function or some other biological deficit. And, just about all these can be corrected without antidepressants. In fact, most people who take antidepressants find that they offer only partial relief, lose effectiveness over time or simply don't work. These drugs also cause side effects such as weight gain and loss of sex drive, and more than half of people who take them quit within months.

In reality, everything that affects the body affects the brain, since it is one of the most vital organs of the body, and everything that affects the brain affects the rest of the body. Simply taking an antidepressant for depression—or Ritalin for ADHD, or an anti-anxiety medication and so forth—fails to take this basic body-mind connection into account. A new paradigm for mental illness must take a wider view of a person, not merely focus on the brain, since there are myriad causes of mental illness. This view should replace the shortsighted approach to treatment where a doctor marks down a diagnostic code on a patient's chart and prescribes the corresponding pill.

Dr. Hyman's Ultramind Solution

There are seven key influences affecting your brain, your memory, attention, mood and behavior—nutrition, hormones, inflammation, digestion, detoxification, energy metabolism and the mind-body connection. When one or more of these are thrown off-kilter, imbalances develop, which can manifest in mental and/or emotional illness. Identifying and addressing imbalances thusly enables the body's natural healing mechanisms to take over, bringing about dramatic improvements in mood, memory, attention, concentration, cognition and other brain functions.

A three-pronged strategy for brain wellness: My book, *The Ultramind Solution: Fix Your Broken Brain by Healing Your Body First*, has quizzes to help identify which of your seven underlying systems isn't working…suggestions on how to fix the underlying problem causing the imbalance…and ways to nourish all these aspects so they can function optimally as an integrated system. Here is a brief look at how each of the seven key systems affects mental health, and what you can do to help keep them in balance.

•**Are you eating right?** Inadequate nutrition is at the root of many illnesses, both mental and physical. If your diet is loaded with fatty fast foods, processed foods and refined carbohydrates (e.g., white bread and pasta) you're not only missing the nutrients your brain requires to function properly, but also creating other chemical imbalances. To restore balance, eat a diet based on a variety of whole, unprocessed foods.

•**Is there a hormonal issue?** Improper diet is among the factors that can lead to a hormone imbalance—specifically, eating sugar and refined carbohydrates causes the body to pump out an overload of the hormone insulin into the bloodstream. Too much insulin can cause mood swings and behavior disturbances such as depression, anxiety, panic attacks and insomnia. Other hormonal imbalances are caused by swings in sex hormones, which can be a natural result of aging, or an improperly functioning thyroid gland, etc. See your physician to identify and treat hormonal issues.

•**Do you need to cool down inflammation?** If the body is inflamed, the brain is too. Brain inflammation is implicated in nearly every brain disease, from Alzheimer's to autism to depression to schizophrenia. Sources of inflammation include refined carbohydrates, food allergens, stress and anxiety—but on the bright side, these are all fixable problems. In addition to eating healthier whole foods, getting plenty of omega-3 fatty acids, and taking steps to control stress, you can also add anti-inflammatory herbs such as turmeric, ginger and rosemary to your diet.

•**Is there a digestive problem?** One of the most powerful ways you can fix your brain is to fix your gut. For example, if your digestive enzymes malfunction, undigested gluten from wheat or casein from milk can harm brain function. Strategies to resolve digestive problems might include eliminating food allergens, considering digestive enzymes and taking probiotics to bring digestive colonies of microbes back into proper balance.

•**Do you need to detox?** Toxic chemicals in the environment such as mercury and lead underlie many neurological diseases. Limit exposure to these toxins to the greatest degree possible. For example, do not eat (or rarely eat) large fish such as swordfish or tuna that is likely to contain higher levels of mercury. If you live in an older house, be sure the water and paint are not contaminated with lead.

•**How's your energy metabolism?** Mitochondria are the miniature energy factories in your body's cells, including those in the brain. The single most important thing you can do to support your mitochondria and boost your energy is to exercise. For energy problems specifically related to stress, toxicity or aging, prescribe supplements such as Acetyl-L-Carnitine, Alpha-lipoic acid, Coenzyme Q10, magnesium, riboflavin and niacin.

•**Are you stressed out?** Closely examine your life. Stress robs you of energy, so take action to more effectively manage it. For instance, make a promise to yourself that this week you will eliminate one thing that causes anxiety and add one that helps you heal and thrive.

Drugs can provide a temporary fix for brain problems, but these are not the long-term solution. As usual, it takes more work than popping a pill, but in the long run a healthy mind and body are worth it.

How to Help Your Brain Heal

Laurie Steelsmith, ND, a licensed naturopathic physician and acupuncturist in private practice in Honolulu and author of *Natural Cures for Women*. DrSteelsmith.com

News stories about concussions have brought this brain injury to the top of our minds—their number doubled between 2005 and 2012 among young athletes (according to a recent study published in *American Journal of Sports and Medicine*), and researchers are looking closely at a pattern of deadly brain disease in former NFL players, trying to discern whether a history of concussions plays a role in its development.

But don't make the mistake of thinking this is a problem only for those playing sports. The truth is that a concussion can be the result of banging your head on a piece of furniture, being in a minor car accident or even tripping over your dog in a dark hallway and bumping your head against the wall. About one million concussions occur in the US each year, according to reports of hospital admissions, and there are likely many more people who have them and don't seek help—in short, we're all at risk.

There has been some fascinating research based on work done with soldiers who had suffered brain injuries. It concluded that one of the most important things to do for someone who has suffered a concussion (or a far more serious traumatic brain injury) is to feed him or her as soon as possible. It seems that making sure patients get at least 50% of their usual calorie intake within 24 hours—including a higher-than-usual amount of protein, which should be continued for two weeks—is vital to healing. A healthy diet makes sense. But what other natural treatments might help heal a hurting brain?

What You Need to Know

First, it's important to review what we should know about concussion, which is like a bruise that results from your brain colliding with your skull. Anyone who has had a blow to the head should consider himself at risk, most especially if there was even a momentary loss of consciousness.

Other signs of concussion: Headache, nausea, difficulty concentrating and/ or short-term memory loss. One or more of these symptoms should trigger a call to your doctor, who will determine if further testing is required.

Naturopathic medicine can offer natural ways to help the tissues heal after a concussion. *Here are the most effective natural remedies...*

•**Load up on antioxidants.** Eat a healthy diet with abundant protein (as mentioned above) and also eat lots of blueberries during the two weeks following the injury.

The reason: Blueberries contain potent flavonoid antioxidants that help to strengthen blood vessel walls, including in the brain. Supplement the fruit's antioxidants by taking up to 3,000 mg a day of vitamin C, which also helps reduce the oxidative stress in the brain associated with head trauma. Buffered powder (vitamin C combined with small amounts of calcium, magnesium and potassium) is most easily absorbed—mix the powder with juice.

•**Drink fluids.** Make sure the body is well-hydrated, as that allows the brain to heal more quickly.

How much to drink: Drink one ounce of fluid (nonalcoholic and preferably noncaffeinated—water is best) per day per two pounds of body weight, so a person who weighs 100 pounds should drink 50 ounces over the course of the day for the critical two weeks.

•**Take arnica** (*Arnica montana*). You are probably familiar with arnica cream, made from a plant that has served medicinal purposes for more than 500 years and used for sore muscles, sprains and bruises. But arnica also comes in the form of homeopathic pellets, which help to expedite healing of bruised brain tissue. Place three homeopathic arnica 30c pellets (available at health stores and online) under your tongue within 15 minutes of the trauma or as soon as you can get them. Continue this dosage every hour for the rest of the day, reducing frequency on the second, third and fourth days to three doses—one in the morning, one at lunch and one in the evening.

•**Double dose of fish oil—fast.** While the general recommendation for most people is to take one to two grams daily of high-potency fish oil, it is a good idea for people who have suffered head injuries to take up to four grams as quickly as possible after the injury and to continue taking four grams once daily for up to seven days afterward. This advice is based on an animal study from West Virginia University School of Medicine reported in the Journal of Neurosurgery, which demonstrated that taking high-potency fish oil that contained large amounts of the omega-3 fatty acids EPA and DHA (such as Nordic Naturals Omega-3D, which contains 745 mg EPA and 500 mg DHA per one-teaspoon serving), can assist in healing concussion. This will help decrease brain inflammation and with it the fogginess, memory loss and headaches that are often a part of concussion.

Note: If there is evidence of bleeding in your brain (see below), do not take fish oil.

Danger Zone

It is important to realize that the danger zone following a concussion can last up to 48 hours, with the first 24 hours being the most critical. The danger is that bleeding will occur in the brain (especially likely if a person is taking an anticoagulant medication such as warfarin) or that a blood clot can form. *The following symptoms should be seen as a medical emergency, warranting a call to 9-1-1 and a visit to the emergency department of the nearest hospital...*

- **A headache that gets continually worse**
- **Vomiting**
- **Slurred speech**
- **One pupil larger than the other or other visual disturbances**
- **Change in sleeping pattern—such as sleeping more than normal**
- **Seizure**
- **Confusion and restlessness**
- **Amnesia**

Luckily, severe problems are quite rare. Most concussions are much less threatening, and most people can heal safely and completely at home.

CHAPTER 5

Stroke Stoppers

Stroke: You Can Do Much More to Protect Yourself

Ralph L. Sacco, MD, chairman of neurology, the Olemberg Family Chair in Neurological Disorders and the Miller Professor of Neurology, Epidemiology and Public Health, Human Genetics and Neurosurgery at the Miller School of Medicine at the University of Miami.

N o one likes to think about having a stroke. But maybe you should.

The grim reality: Stroke strikes nearly 795,000 Americans each year and is the leading cause of disability.

Now for the remarkable part: About 80% of strokes can be prevented. You may think that you've heard it all when it comes to preventing strokes—it's about controlling your blood pressure, eating a good diet and getting some exercise, right? Actually, that's only part of what you can be doing to protect yourself. *Surprising recent findings on stroke—and the latest advice on how to avoid it…*

•**Even "low" high blood pressure is a red flag.** High blood pressure—a reading of 140/90 mmHg or higher—is widely known to increase one's odds of having a stroke. But even slight elevations in blood pressure may also be a problem.

An important recent study that looked at data from more than half a million patients found that those with blood pressure readings that were just slightly higher than a normal reading of 120/80 mmHg were more likely to have a stroke.

Any increase in blood pressure is worrisome. In fact, the risk for a stroke or heart attack doubles for each 20-point rise in systolic (the top number) pressure above 115/75 mmHg—and for each 10-point rise in diastolic (the bottom number) pressure.

My advice: Don't wait for your doctor to recommend treatment if your blood pressure is even a few points higher than normal. Tell him/her that you are concerned. Lifestyle changes—such as getting adequate exercise, avoiding excess alcohol and maintaining a healthful diet—often reverse slightly elevated blood pressure. Blood pressure consistently above 140/90 mmHg generally requires medication.

•**Sleep can be dangerous.** People who are sleep deprived—generally defined as getting less than six hours of sleep per night—are at increased risk for stroke.

What most people don't realize is that getting too much sleep is also a problem. When researchers at the University of Cambridge tracked the sleep habits of nearly 10,000 people over a 10-year period, they found that those who slept more than eight hours a night were 46% more likely to have a stroke than those who slept six to eight hours.

It is possible that people who spend less/more time sleeping have other, unrecognized conditions that affect both sleep and stroke risk.

Example: Sleep apnea, a breathing disorder that interferes with sleep, causes an increase in blood pressure that can lead to stroke. Meanwhile, sleeping too much can be a symptom of depression—another stroke risk factor.

My advice: See a doctor if you tend to wake up unrefreshed...are a loud snorer...or often snort or thrash while you sleep. You may have sleep apnea. If you sleep too much, also talk to your doctor to see if you are suffering from depression or some other condition that may increase your stroke risk.

What's the sweet spot for nightly shut-eye? When it comes to stroke risk, it's six to eight hours per night.

•**What you drink matters, too.** A Mediterranean-style diet—plenty of whole grains, legumes, nuts, fish, produce and olive oil—is perhaps the best diet going when it comes to minimizing stroke risk. A recent study concluded that about 30% of strokes could be prevented if people simply switched to this diet.

But there's more you can do. Research has found that people who drank six cups of green or black tea a day were 42% less likely to have strokes than people who did not drink tea. With three daily cups, risk dropped by 21%.

The antioxidant *epigallocatechin gallate* or the amino acid *L-theanine* may be responsible.

●**Emotional stress shouldn't be pooh-poohed.** If you're prone to angry outbursts, don't assume it's no big deal. Emotional stress triggers the release of cortisol, adrenaline and other so-called stress hormones that can increase blood pressure and heart rate, leading to stroke.

In one study, about 30% of stroke patients had heightened negative emotions (such as anger) in the two hours preceding the stroke.

My advice: Don't ignore your mental health—especially anger (it's often a sign of depression, a potent stroke risk factor). If you're suffering from "negative" emotions, exercise regularly, try relaxation strategies (such as meditation) and don't hesitate to get professional help.

●**Be alert for subtle signs of stroke.** The acronym "FAST" helps people identify signs of stroke. "F" stands for facial drooping—does one side of the face droop or is it numb? Is the person's smile uneven? "A" stands for arm weakness—ask the person to raise both arms. Does one arm drift downward? "S" stands for speech difficulty—is speech slurred? Is the person unable to speak or hard to understand? Can he/she repeat a simple sentence such as, "The sky is blue" correctly? "T" stands for time—if a person shows any of these symptoms (even if they go away), call 911 immediately. Note the time so that you know when symptoms first appeared.

But stroke can also cause one symptom that isn't widely known—a loss of touch sensation. This can occur if a stroke causes injury to the parts of the brain that detect touch. If you suddenly can't "feel" your fingers or toes—or have trouble with simple tasks such as buttoning a shirt—you could be having a stroke. You might notice that you can't feel temperatures or that you can't feel it when your feet touch the floor.

It's never normal to lose your sense of touch for an unknown reason—or to have unexpected difficulty seeing, hearing and/or speaking. Get to an emergency room!

Also important: If you think you're having a stroke, don't waste time calling your regular doctor. Call an ambulance, and ask to be taken to the nearest hospital with a primary stroke center. You'll get much better care than you would at a regular hospital emergency room.

A meta-analysis found that there were 21% fewer deaths among patients treated at stroke centers, and the surviving patients had faster recoveries and fewer stroke-related complications.

My advice: If you have any stroke risk factors, including high blood pressure, diabetes or elevated cholesterol, find out now which hospitals in your area have stroke centers. To find one near you, go to HospitalMaps.heart.org.

Uncommon Stroke Risks You Need to Know

Louis R. Caplan, MD, senior neurologist at Beth Israel Deaconess Medical Center and a professor of neurology at Harvard Medical School, both in Boston. He has written or edited more than 40 books, including *Stroke* (*What Do I Do Now?*) and *Navigating the Complexities of Stroke.*

What if there were more to preventing a stroke than keeping your blood pressure under control…getting regular exercise…watching your body weight…and not smoking? Researchers are now discovering that there is.

New thinking: While most stroke sufferers say that "it just came out of the blue," an increasing body of evidence shows that these potentially devastating "brain attacks" can be caused by conditions that you might ordinarily think are completely unrelated.

Once you're aware of these "hidden" risk factors—and take the necessary steps to prevent or control them—you can improve your odds of never having a stroke. *Recently discovered stroke risk factors…*

Inflammatory Bowel Disease

Both Crohn's disease and ulcerative colitis can severely damage the large or small intestine. But that is not the only risk. Among patients who have either one of these conditions, known as inflammatory bowel disease (IBD), stroke is the third most common cause of death, according to some estimates.

During flare-ups, patients with IBD have elevated blood levels of substances that trigger clots—the cause of most strokes. A Harvard study, for example, found that many IBD patients have high levels of C-reactive protein (CRP), an inflammatory marker that has been linked to atherosclerotic lesions, damaged areas in blood vessels that can lead to stroke-causing clots in the brain.

If you have IBD: Ask your doctor what you can do to reduce your risk for blood clots and inflammation. Some patients with IBD can't take aspirin or other anticlotting drugs because these medications frequently cause intestinal bleeding. Instead of aspirin, you might be advised to take an autoimmune medication such as *azathioprine* (Azasan, Imuran), which suppresses the immune system and reduces inflammation. During flare-ups, some patients are given steroids to further reduce inflammation.

Side effects, including nausea and vomiting with azathioprine use and weight gain and increased blood pressure with steroid use, usually can be minimized by taking the lowest possible dose.

Some physicians recommend omega-3 fish oil supplements for IBD, which are less likely to cause side effects. Ask your doctor whether these supplements (and what dose) are right for you.

Important: Strokes tend to occur in IBD patients when inflammation is most severe. To check inflammatory markers, CRP levels and *erythrocyte sedimentation rate* (ESR) can be measured. Tests for clotting include *fibrinogen* and *d-dimer*. The results of these tests will help determine the course of the patient's IBD treatment.

Migraines

Migraine headaches accompanied by *auras* (characterized by the appearance of flashing lights or other visual disturbances) are actually a greater risk factor for stroke than obesity, smoking or diabetes (see page 94), according to a startling study presented at a recent annual meeting of the American Academy of Neurology.

When researchers use MRIs to examine blood vessels in the brain, they find more tiny areas of arterial damage in patients who have migraines with auras than in those who don't get migraines. (Research shows that there is no link between stroke and migraines that aren't accompanied by auras.)

If you have migraines with auras: Reduce your risk by controlling other stroke risk factors—don't smoke...lose weight if you're overweight...and control cholesterol levels.

Also: Women under age 50 who have migraines (with or without auras) may be advised to not use combined-hormone forms of birth control pills—they slightly increase risk for stroke. In addition, patients who have migraines with auras should not take beta-blockers, such as *propranolol* (Inderal), or the triptan drugs, such as *sumatriptan* (Imitrex), commonly used for migraine headaches. These drugs can also increase stroke risk. For frequent migraines with auras, I often prescribe the blood pressure drug *verapamil* (Calan) and a daily 325-mg aspirin. Ask your doctor for advice.

Rheumatoid Arthritis

Rheumatoid arthritis, unlike the common "wear-and-tear" variety (osteoarthritis), is an autoimmune disease that not only causes inflammation in the joints but may also trigger it in the heart, blood vessels and other parts of the body.

Arterial inflammation increases the risk for blood clots, heart attack and stroke. In fact, patients with severe rheumatoid arthritis were almost twice as likely to have a stroke as those without the disease, according to a study published in *Arthritis Care & Research*.

If you have rheumatoid arthritis: Work with your rheumatologist to manage flare-ups and reduce systemic inflammation. Your doctor will probably recommend that you take one or more anti-inflammatory painkillers, such as *ibuprofen* (Motrin). In addition, he/she might prescribe a *disease-modifying antirheumatic drug* (DMARD), such as *methotrexate* (Trexall), to slow the progression of the disease—and the increased risk for stroke. Fish oil also may be prescribed to reduce joint tenderness.

Strokes tend to occur in rheumatoid arthritis patients when inflammation is peaking. Ask your doctor if you should have the inflammation tests (CRP and ESR) mentioned in the IBD section.

Diabetes

If you have diabetes or diabetes risk factors—such as obesity, a sedentary lifestyle or a family history of diabetes—protect yourself. People with diabetes are up to four times more likely to have a stroke than those without it.

High blood sugar in people with diabetes damages blood vessels throughout the body, including in the brain. The damage can lead to both *ischemic* (clot-related) and *hemorrhagic* (bleeding) strokes.

If you have diabetes: Work closely with your doctor. Patients who achieve good glucose control with oral medications and/or insulin are much less likely to suffer from vascular damage.

Also important: Lose weight if you need to. Weight loss combined with exercise helps your body metabolize blood sugar more efficiently. In those with mild diabetes, weight loss combined with exercise may restore normal blood sugar levels…and can reduce complications and the need for medications in those with more serious diabetes.

Clotting Disorders

Any condition that affects the blood's normal clotting functions can increase risk for stroke.

Examples: Thrombocytosis (excessive platelets in the blood)…an elevated *hematocrit* (higher-than-normal percentage of red blood cells)…or *Factor V Leiden* (an inherited tendency to form blood clots). Clotting tests (fibrinogen and d-dimer) are recommended for these disorders.

If you have a clotting disorder: Ask your doctor what you can do to protect yourself from stroke.

Example: If you have an elevated hematocrit, your doctor might advise you to drink more fluids.

This is particularly important for older adults, who tend to drink less later in the day because they don't want to get up at night to urinate. I recommend that these patients drink approximately 80 ounces of noncaffeine-containing fluids during the day, stopping by 7 pm. People who don't take in enough fluids can develop "thick" blood that impedes circulation—and increases the risk for clots.

Artery Inflammation: Six Simple, Lifesaving Tests

Bradley Bale, MD, medical director, Grace Clinic Heart Health Program, Lubbock, Texas, and cofounder, Heart Attack & Stroke Prevention Center, Spokane. He is co-author, with Amy Doneen, ARNP, and Lisa Collier Cool, of *Beat the Heart Attack Gene: The Revolutionary Plan to Prevent Heart Disease, Stroke and Diabetes.*

A fire could be smoldering inside your arteries…a type of fire that could erupt at any moment, triggering a heart attack or stroke. In fact, the fire could be building right this minute and you wouldn't even know it. That's because the usual things doctors look at when gauging cardiovascular risk—cholesterol, blood pressure, blood sugar, weight—can all appear to be fine even when your arteries are dangerously hot.

What does work to detect hot arteries? A set of six simple, inexpensive and readily available blood and urine tests.

Problem: Few doctors order these tests, and few patients know enough to ask for them. Without the warnings these tests provide, patients often have no way of knowing just how great their risk is for heart attack or stroke and whether or not their preventive treatments are working—until it's too late. *Here's how to protect yourself...*

The Body's Army on Attack

Hot arteries are not actually hot (as in very warm)—instead, in this case "hot" refers to the effects of chronic inflammation. Why call them hot, then? Chronic arterial inflammation can put you on the fast track to developing vascular disease by speeding up the aging of your arteries. It's so dangerous to the arterial lining that it's worse than having high LDL cholesterol. And if your arteries are already clogged with plaque—which acts as kindling for a heart attack or stroke—inflammation is what lights the match.

Inflammation in the body isn't always bad, of course. In fact, it's an important aspect of healing. When something in your body is under attack, the immune system sends in troops of white blood cells to repair and fight off the attacker, and temporary inflammation results. That's why when you cut yourself, for example, you'll see swelling at the site of the injury—it's a sign that your white blood cells are at work for your benefit.

But: When an attack against your body persists (for instance, as occurs when you have an ongoing infection of the gums), your white blood cells continue to drive inflammation. When it turns chronic, inflammation becomes highly damaging to many tissues, including the arteries.

Normally, the *endothelium* (lining of the arteries) serves as a protective barrier between blood and the deeper layers of the arterial wall. However, when that lining is inflamed, it can't function well and it gets sticky, almost like flypaper, trapping white blood cells on their way through the body. The inflamed endothelium becomes leaky, too, allowing LDL "bad" cholesterol to penetrate into the wall of the artery. The white blood cells then gobble up the cholesterol, forming fatty streaks that ultimately turn into plaque, a condition called atherosclerosis. Then when the plaque itself becomes inflamed, it can rupture, tearing through the endothelium into the channel of the artery where blood flows. This material triggers the formation of a blood clot—a clot that could end up blocking blood flow to the heart or brain.

The 6-Part Fire Panel

Just as firefighters have ways of determining whether a blaze is hiding within the walls of a building, certain tests can reveal whether inflammation is lurking within the walls of your arteries. I use a set of six tests that I call the "fire panel." Each reveals different risk factors and, for several of the tests, too-high scores can have more than one cause—so it's important to get all six tests, not just one or two.

The fire panel can identify people at risk for developing atherosclerosis... reveal whether patients who already have atherosclerosis have dangerously hot arteries that could lead to a heart attack or stroke...and evaluate patients who have survived a heart attack or stroke to see whether their current treatments are working to reduce the inflammation that threatens their lives. Your individual test results will help determine your most appropriate course of treatment.

I recommend that all adults have this panel of tests done at least every 12 months—or every three to six months for patients at high risk for heart attack or stroke. All of these tests are readily available...are inexpensive and usually covered by insurance...and can be ordered by your regular doctor. *Here are the six tests...*

•**F2 Isoprostanes.** My nickname for this blood test is the "lifestyle lie detector" because it reveals whether or not patients are practicing heart-healthy habits. The test, which measures a biomarker of oxidative stress, helps determine how fast your body's cells are oxidizing, or breaking down. According to one study, people who have the highest levels of F2 isoprostanes are nine times more likely to have blockages in their coronary arteries than people with the lowest levels.

The score you want: A normal score is less than 0.86 ng/L...an optimal score is less than 0.25 ng/L.

•**Fibrinogen.** An abnormally high level of this sticky, fibrous protein in your blood can contribute to the formation of clots...it's also a marker of inflammation. One study divided people into four groups (quartiles) based on their fibrinogen levels and found that stroke risk rose by nearly 50% for each quartile. High fibrinogen is particularly dangerous for people who also have high blood pressure because both conditions damage the blood vessel lining and make it easier for plaque to burrow inside.

Normal range: 440 mg/dL or lower.

•**High-Sensitivity C-Reactive Protein (hs-CRP).** Your liver produces C-reactive protein, and the amount of it in your blood rises when there is inflammation in your body—so an elevated hs-CRP level generally is considered a precursor to cardiovascular disease. The large-scale Harvard Women's Health

Study cited this test as being more accurate than cholesterol in predicting risk for cardiovascular disease...while another study of women found that those with high scores were up to four times more likely to have a heart attack or stroke than women with lower scores. A high hs-CRP score is especially worrisome for a person with a large waist. Excess belly fat often is a sign of insulin resistance (in which cells don't readily accept insulin), a condition that further magnifies heart attack and stroke risk.

The score you're aiming for: Under 1.0 mg/L is normal...0.5 mg/L is optimal.

•**Microalbumin/Creatinine Urine Ratio (MACR).** This test looks for albumin in the urine. Albumin is a large protein molecule that circulates in the blood and shouldn't spill from capillaries in the kidneys into the urine, so its presence suggests dysfunction of the endothelium. Though this test provides valuable information about arterial wall health, doctors rarely use it for this purpose.

Important: New evidence shows that MACR levels that have traditionally been considered "normal" can signal increased risk for cardiovascular events.

Optimal ratios, according to the latest research: 7.5 or lower for women and 4.0 or lower for men.

•**Lipoprotein-Associated Phospholipase A-2 (Lp-PLA2).** This enzyme in the blood is attached to LDL cholesterol and rises when artery walls become inflamed. Recent research suggests that it plays a key role in the atherosclerosis disease process, contributing to the formation of plaque as well as to the plaque's vulnerability to rupture. People with periodontal (gum) disease are especially likely to have elevated Lp-PLA2 scores—chronic inflammation can start in unhealthy gums and, from there, spread to the arteries.

Normal range: Less than 200 ng/mL.

•**Myeloperoxidase (MPO).** This immune system enzyme normally is found at elevated levels only at the site of an infection. When it is elevated in the bloodstream, it must be assumed that it's due to significant inflammation in the artery walls and leaking through the endothelium. This is a very bad sign. MPO produces numerous oxidants that make all cholesterol compounds, including HDL "good" cholesterol, more inflammatory. If your blood levels of MPO are high, HDL goes rogue and joins the gang of inflammatory thugs. It also interacts with another substance in the bloodstream to produce an acid that can eat holes in blood vessel walls. Smokers are particularly prone to high MPO levels.

Normal range: Less than 420 pmol/L.

How to Put Out the Fires

While the "fire panel" tests above may seem exotic, the solution to the hot artery problem, for most of us, is not. That's because the best way to combat chronic inflammation is simply to maintain a healthful lifestyle. You just have to do it! *Key factors include...*

- Following a heart-healthy Mediterranean- style diet.
- Managing stress.
- Getting plenty of exercise.
- Guarding against insulin resistance.
- Taking good care of your teeth and gums.
- Not smoking.

In some cases, lifestyle changes alone are enough to quell the flames of chronic inflammation and to put your arteries on the road to recovery. In other cases, patients also need medication such as statins and/or dietary supplements such as niacin and fish oil. Either way, the good news is that once you shut the inflammation off, the body has a chance to heal whatever disease and damage has occurred—so you're no longer on the fast track to a heart attack or stroke.

More Magnesium, Please!

Roger Bonomo, MD, neurologist in private practice, stroke specialist and former director, Stroke Center, Lenox Hill Hospital, New York City.

Consuming an additional 100 mg of magnesium a day may reduce your risk for stroke by 9%. And magnesium isn't an expensive drug with side effects—it's a natural mineral that's already in many of the foods we eat. Most of us, especially those of us at high risk for stroke, high blood pressure or diabetes—would benefit from eating more magnesium-rich foods, such as...

- **Pumpkin seeds** (191 mg per ¼ cup)
- **Almonds** (160 mg per 2 oz.)
- **Spinach** (156 mg per cup)
- **Cashews** (148 mg per 2 oz.)
- **White beans** (134 mg per cup)
- **Artichokes** (97 mg per one large artichoke)
- **Brown rice** (84 mg per cup)
- **Shrimp** (39 mg per 4 oz.)

You can also supercharge your cooking with magnesium if you use oat bran (221 mg per cup) and buckwheat flour (301 mg per cup).

Should anyone be concerned about overdosing on magnesium? It's hard to eat too much magnesium. If we do, our kidneys excrete the extra through urine, so only those with kidney failure need to make sure they don't consume too much.

How Art Safeguards Your Brain Against Stroke

Ercole Vellone, PhD, RN, an assistant professor of nursing science in the School of Nursing at University of Rome "Tor Vergata" in Italy, and lead author of a study on stroke presented at a recent meeting of the Council on Cardiovascular Nursing and Allied Professions of the European Society of Cardiology.

As we stroll through a favorite museum, listen to some great music or splurge on theater tickets, we could be benefiting our brains—in a way that is far more significant and surprising than the simple fun such activities provide. Why? Because when it comes to recovering from stroke, a recent study suggests, art lovers enjoy an important advantage. This is big news, given that stroke is the leading cause of disability among adults in the U.S.

Researchers asked 192 stroke survivors whether they liked or did not like art, such as painting, music and theater. Of the participants, 105 said that they did like the arts...the other 87 had no particular interest in art (the clinical condition of both groups was similar).

Findings: After adjusting for participants' prestroke health status, researchers found that, regardless of the gravity of the strokes, patients who regarded art as an "integrated part of their former lifestyle" tended to...

• **Have more energy.**

• **Experience less difficulty walking.**

• **Feel calmer, happier, less depressed and less anxious.**

• **Have better memory.**

Coffee Reduces Stroke Risk

Drinking one or more cups of caffeinated or decaffeinated coffee daily was associated with a 22% to 25% reduction in stroke risk.

Theory: Coffee beans contain antioxidants and other disease-fighting chemicals that may reduce inflammation and improve insulin activity, which lowers blood glucose levels and reduces stroke risk.

Susanna C. Larsson, PhD, a nutritional epidemiologist, Institute of Environmental Medicine, Karolinska Institute, Stockholm, Sweden, and lead researcher of a study of 34,670 women, published in *Stroke*.

•**Show superior communication abilities** (such as speaking, comprehension and correctly naming people and objects).

•**Have better general health.**

Why art is smart: Researchers suggested that art may create long-term changes to the brain that help it recover after a trauma such as a stroke.

Not a lifelong lover of the arts? It is unclear whether nurturing a new appreciation for art later in life—or even after a stroke has already occurred—also has recovery benefits. But it might! So why not take yourself to a play, concert or gallery more often? Your brain may someday be the better for it.

Dietary Fiber Cuts Stroke Risk

Victoria J. Burley, PhD, associate professor in nutritional epidemiology at University of Leeds, England, and coauthor of an analysis of eight studies, published in *Stroke*.

For every 7 grams (g) of fiber eaten daily, the risk for a first-time stroke decreased by 7%, in a recent analysis. One serving of whole-wheat pasta or two servings of fruits and vegetables contain about 7 g of fiber. Other top fiber sources include brown rice, spelt, quinoa and other whole-grain foods… almonds and other nuts…lentils and other dried beans.

Recommended daily fiber intake: People age 50 or younger, 38 g (men) and 25 g (women)…over age 50, 30 g (men) and 21 g (women).

Animal Protein for Stroke Prevention

Xinfeng Liu, MD, PhD, professor and chairman, department of neurology, Jinling Hospital, Nanjing University School of Medicine, China. His study was published in *Neurology*.

You already know what not to eat to protect yourself from stroke, so you stay away from foods that are high in salt and artery-clogging fats. And you probably know that you should be eating lots of fruits, vegetables and whole grains for their fiber and healthful antioxidants. But there's another nutrient that you need for stroke protection. Protein—yes, protein. And here's the surprise—although nuts, beans and grains are all protein sources known for helping heart health, the results of a recent study suggest that a certain kind of animal protein may be the best for stroke protection.

You're probably thinking that makes no sense. Many studies have shown that protein-rich diets, particularly diets in which the protein mostly comes from animals, are not beneficial for stroke prevention. At the same time, other studies have shown that protein-rich diets can reduce stroke risk.

Researchers from China who tried to make sense of conflicting studies about protein and stroke risk found that people whose diets included a moderate to moderately high amount of protein—particularly animal protein (up to 2.19 ounces per day compared with the average US recommended amount of 1.6 to 2 ounces of protein from any source)—were less likely to have a stroke than people who included only a little bit of protein in their diets. In looking at a group of studies that, in total, included 254,489 people, the researchers discovered that people who ate the most protein from any source had a 20% lower risk of stroke compared with those who consumed the least protein. Also, interestingly, the more protein eaten from any source, the lower the risk of stroke. That is, for every 0.7 ounces more of protein (moderately) consumed, stroke risk dropped by 26%.

In studies that specifically looked at either animal protein or vegetable protein, the researchers discovered that eating more, rather than less, animal protein reduced risk by 29% and eating more, rather than less, vegetable protein reduced risk by 12%. The range between high and low consumption in the studies on vegetable protein wasn't that wide, though, which may be why a larger difference in stroke risk reduction wasn't seen in them.

The Best Source of Protein

Here's the most valuable takeaway from the meta-study—the greatest benefit for stroke protection, by far, seemed to come from getting animal protein from fish.

When the Chinese researchers looked more closely at the individual scientific studies, they noticed something striking about cultural and regional differences that put the puzzle about protein and stroke risk all together for them. Studies from Japan—a country in which fish consumption is particularly high—showed that people who ate the most protein had half the stroke risk of people who ate the least. And a research paper from Sweden—another country big on fish-eating—showed that stroke risk was reduced by 26% in higher consumers of protein. Compare these risk numbers to the one pooled from four studies from the United States, whose residents, on average, get the least amount of their protein from fish. Stroke risk reduction from higher protein consumption was only 9%.

How does protein reduce stroke risk? One theory is that it does so by lowering blood pressure, a well-known risk factor for stroke.

> ### Optimism Prevents Strokes
>
> Each "unit increase" in optimism—the general expectation that more good than bad will happen in the future—reduced stroke risk by 9% over the next two years in a recent study. And each unit increase in sense of purpose reduced heart attack risk by 27% over the same period.
>
> *Possible reason:* People with purpose and a positive outlook may take better care of themselves.
>
> The late Christopher Peterson, PhD, professor of psychology, University of Michigan, Ann Arbor, and coauthor of two studies published in *Stroke*.

Red meat, poultry, fish and dairy all contain L-arginine, an amino acid that our bodies convert to nitric oxide. Nitric oxide causes blood vessels to open wider, which improves blood flow and reduces blood pressure. But this good effect might be countered by the types of fat (and cholesterol) in red meat and dairy. This is why fish, which contains other heart-healthy nutrients such as omega-3 fatty acids, looks like the better choice.

This study makes a strong case that fish should be our main source of protein. The Mediterranean diet—a diet high in whole grains, vegetables, olive oil, fish and fruit and low in red meat—is beneficial for stroke reduction. So, if you're already fortifying your diet with vegetables and protein and especially substituting fish for red meat, you're doing it right. If not, consider making this heart-healthy change now.

Most Important Meal

Study of 82,772 people led by researchers at Osaka University Graduate School of Medicine, Japan, published in *Stroke*.

D id you know that eating breakfast may lower stroke risk? People who never ate breakfast had a higher risk for hemorrhagic (bleeding in the brain) strokes than people who ate breakfast daily.

Possible reason: High blood pressure is a major risk factor for hemorrhagic stroke. Eating breakfast is associated with a drop in blood pressure.

A Grapefruit a Day Helps Keep Stroke Away

Kathryn M. Rexrode, MD, MPH, physician, division of preventive medicine, Brigham and Women's Hospital, and assistant professor of medicine, Harvard Medical School, both in Boston.

Mmm, citrus. There's nothing like a refreshing orange, a tangy tangerine or a sweet pink grapefruit. It really does taste like sunshine.

But these juicy fruits aren't just delicious—they may actually help you ward off a stroke, according to recent research.

And you may be surprised to hear that it's not because of the vitamin C…

Honing in on Flavonoids

A zillion studies have shown the health benefits of eating fruit, including studies that have shown that people who eat five or more servings of fruits and vegetables have a 25% lower risk for stroke (both ischemic and hemorrhagic) compared with those who eat three or fewer servings. Researchers have suspected that flavonoids, antioxidant compounds found in many fruits and vegetables, are one key to their power since they reduce inflammation and improve blood vessel function.

But there are six different types of flavonoids found in foods, and each has a subtly different chemical structure. Given the variety, researchers from England, Italy and the US wanted to learn which specific flavonoids and which fruits or vegetables, in particular, are most beneficial for preventing stroke.

More about the study…

The Flavonoid That Came Out On Top

The researchers used information from 70,000 women who were followed for 14 years as part of the Nurses' Health Study. Every two years, the participants completed questionnaires that covered their medical histories and lifestyles. And every four years, the women completed food questionnaires, which asked how much of certain foods and drinks they consumed and how often they consumed them.

The women's diets were analyzed for the six different types of flavonoids, and their medical histories were reviewed for the number and type of strokes that the women had. What they found was that high consumption—more than about 63 milligrams per day of a certain subclass of flavonoids called *flavanones* (the amount found in about one to two servings of citrus per day)—

was associated with a 19% reduced risk for ischemic stroke (the type caused by a clot, not by a bleed), compared with low flavanone consumption (under 13.7 milligrams per day). And this was after adjusting for other stroke risk factors, such as smoking, age, body mass index and others. The other five flavonoids studied reduced stroke risk, too, but not by as much (only by 4% to 13%).

One reason that the flavanones may have been associated with decreased risk for ischemic stroke is that flavanones may inhibit platelet function and clotting factors. The researchers didn't study whether citrus affected risk for hemorrhagic stroke, but it's unlikely that eating citrus would lead to an increased risk for hemorrhagic stroke. It takes a relatively small amount of clotting to cause an ischemic stroke, but, on the other hand, it takes a relatively large amount of excessive bleeding to cause a hemorrhagic stroke.

Although this study, which was published in *Stroke*, looked only at women, there is no reason to think that these findings wouldn't apply to men, too.

Pick Your Citrus

You can get all the flavanones you need (about 63 milligrams) from eating one or two servings of citrus each day. Whole fruits are always better than juices or smoothies, because the bulk of the flavanones are found in the inner membranes of the fruit and the pith or white part of the fruit. The pith is generally removed when the fruit is juiced or cleaned for smoothies.

The USDA provides information about the amount of flavanones in every 100 grams of edible fruit, so to save you the trouble of weighing your fruits, here are estimates of the flavanone content for some common citruses...

- **Grapefruit** (½ of a 4-inch diameter) 47 milligrams
- **Orange** (2⅝ inch diameter) 42 milligrams
- **Tangerine** (2½ inch diameter) 18 milligrams

Supplements are not recommended—sticking to whole fruit is best. And don't overdo it on citrus, or else your stomach or teeth might suffer from the acid. Just a serving or two a day is all you need!

Tomato Sauce Reduces Stroke Risk

Rafael Alexander Ortiz, MD, chief, Neuro-Endovascular Surgery and Interventional Neuroradiology, Lenox Hill Hospital, New York City.

R*ecent finding:* People with the highest blood levels of the antioxidant lycopene had 55% lower risk for stroke than people with the lowest levels. Lycopene is found in tomatoes, red peppers, carrots, papaya and watermelon. It is even more concentrated in cooked tomato products, such as tomato sauce.

Easy Stroke Fighter: Red Peppers

Stéphane Vannier, MD, neurologist, Pontchaillou University Hospital, Rennes, France, from research presented at a recent annual meeting of the American Academy of Neurology.

Eating red peppers and other vitamin C–rich fruits and veggies may reduce your risk for intracerebral hemorrhagic stroke (a blood vessel rupture in the brain). And what's so great about red peppers? At 190 mg per cup, they contain three times more vitamin C than an orange. Other good sources of vitamin C—broccoli and strawberries. Researchers believe that this vitamin may reduce stroke risk by regulating blood pressure and strengthening collagen, which promotes healthy blood vessels.

Tasty Treat to Stop Stroke

Sarah Sahib, researcher at McMaster University, Hamilton, Ontario, Canada, lead author of an analysis of studies on chocolate and stroke.

In one study, people who ate one serving of chocolate a week were 22% less likely to have a stroke than those who ate no chocolate. In another study, people who ate 50 grams (1.75 ounces) of chocolate per week were 46% less likely to die following a stroke than those who ate no chocolate.

Possible reason: Chocolate is a rich source of antioxidants that may protect against stroke.

Olive Oil Can Keep Strokes Away

Cécilia Samieri, PhD, researcher, department of epidemiology, Université Bordeaux Segalen, France, and leader of two studies on olive oil consumption and stroke risk, published in *Neurology.*

People who consistently added olive oil to their food in cooking and salad dressings were 41% less likely to suffer from an ischemic stroke than people who did not use olive oil, a recent study found. An ischemic stroke, in which blood flow to a part of the brain is blocked, is the most common kind of stroke.

Folic Acid Cuts Stroke Risk

Meir Stampfer, MD, DrPH, professor of medicine at Harvard Medical School, Boston, and coauthor of an editorial published in *JAMA.*

According to a large study, supplements of the B vitamin decrease incidence of a first stroke in people with high blood pressure by 21%. People with normal blood pressure are likely to benefit, too. A standard daily multivitamin should provide adequate folic acid.

Better: Getting the vitamin from food, especially broccoli, beans (cooked from dried) and dark, leafy greens.

Also: Enriched grain products.

A Single Drink Doubles Your Stroke Risk

Murray A. Mittleman, MD, DrPH, director of the Cardiovascular Epidemiology Research Unit, Beth Israel Deaconess Medical Center, Harvard Medical School, Boston, and leader of a study published in *Stroke.*

Stroke risk is doubled in the hour after you have just one alcoholic drink. The heightened risk for ischemic stroke goes away within three hours.

Theory: Alcohol may temporarily raise blood pressure or affect the blood's ability to clot.

Self-defense: Avoid consuming multiple drinks in a short time because this may cause a sharp increase in stroke risk. One drink is defined as 12 ounces of beer, four ounces of wine, 1.5 ounces of 80-proof spirits or one ounce of 100-proof spirits.

Incredible Eggs!

Dominik D. Alexander, PhD, MSPH, principal epidemiologist, EpidStat Institute, Ann Arbor, Michigan.

Eating up to one egg each day cut stroke risk by 12%—without increasing risk for heart disease—a new study of more than 300,000 adults has found.

Theory: Eggs are rich in antioxidants (shown to reduce inflammation) and protein—both of which help lower blood pressure, an important risk factor for stroke.

CHAPTER 6

Brain Fitness

Best Workouts to Keep Your Brain "Buff"

Cynthia R. Green, PhD, a practicing clinical psychologist and the founder and president of Memory Arts, LLC, a brain-health and memory fitness consulting service in Montclair, New Jersey. She is also founding director of the Memory Enhancement Program at the Icahn School of Medicine at Mount Sinai in New York City. She is author of *Your Best Brain Ever: A Complete Guide & Workout.* TotalBrainHealth.com

We all want to keep our brains in top shape. But are crossword puzzles, online classes and the other such activities that we've been hearing about for years the best ways to do that? Not really.

Now: To improve memory and preserve overall cognitive function, the latest research reveals that it takes more than quiet puzzle-solving and streaming lectures.

Even more intriguing: Some activities that we once thought were time wasters may actually help build intellectual capacity and other cognitive functions.

Cynthia R. Green, PhD, a psychologist and a leading brain trainer explained more about the most effective ways to keep your brain "buff"...

A Healthy Brain

The most important steps to keep your brain performing at optimal levels are lifestyle choices...

- **Getting aerobic exercise** (at least 150 minutes per week).
- **Maintaining a healthy body weight.**
- **Not smoking.**

•**Eating a diet that emphasizes fruits and vegetables and is low in refined sugar and white flour**—two of the biggest dietary threats to brain health that have recently been identified by researchers.

Additional benefits are possible with regular brain workouts. In the past, experts thought that nearly any game or activity that challenges you to think would improve your general brain functioning.

What research now tells us: An increasing body of evidence shows that improved memory requires something more—you need to work against a clock. Games with a time limit force you to think quickly and with agility. These are the factors that lead to improved memory and mental focus.

Among Dr. Green's favorite brain workouts—aim for at least 30 minutes daily of any combination of the activities below...

Cell Phone Games Are Great for Your Brain

Games on your cell phone are better for your brain than crossword or sudoku puzzles.

Reason: They have a timing component.

As you age, your brain faces more challenges with short-term memory and the cognitive tasks of paying attention and juggling multiple abilities. It's important to challenge these skills, and playing games against a clock provides a better brain workout than puzzles and board games.

Cynthia R. Green, PhD, founder and president of Memory Arts, LLC, a memory fitness and brain-health consulting service in Montclair, New Jersey, and founding director of the Memory Enhancement Program at Mount Sinai School of Medicine in New York City. She is author of *Total Memory Workout: 8 Easy Steps to Maximum Memory Fitness.* TotalBrainHealth.com

Brainy Computer Games

Specialized brain-training computer programs (such as Lumosity, Fit Brains and CogniFit) are no longer the darlings of the health community. Formerly marketed as a fun way to reduce one's risk for dementia, recent evidence has not supported that claim.

These programs do provide, however, a variety of activities that may help improve intellectual performance, attention, memory and mental flexibility. Lumosity and other programs are a good option for people who enjoy a regimented brain workout, including such activities as remembering sequences and ignoring distractions. Monthly prices range from $4.99 to $19.95.

Other options to consider trying...

•**Action video games.** These games were once considered "brain-numbing" activities that kept players from developing intellectual and social skills. Recent research, however, shows that action video games can promote mental focus, flexible thinking,, and decision-making and problem-solving skills. Because these games are timed, they also require quick responses from the players.

Good choices: World of Warcraft, *The Elder Scrolls* and *Guild Wars*, all of which involve role-playing by assuming the identity of various characters to battle foes and complete quests, often with other virtual players. These games are available in DVD format for Mac or PC and with an online subscription for virtual play.

Caveat: An hour or two can be a brain booster, but don't overdo it. Too much role-playing takes you away from real-life interactions.

•**Free brain-boosting computer game for a cause.** At FreeRice.com, you can answer fun and challenging questions in such subjects as English vocabulary, foreign languages, math and humanities. With each correct answer, the United Nations World Food Programme donates 10 grains of rice to a Third World country. To date, players have "earned" a total of nearly 100 billion grains of rice—enough to create more than 10 million meals.

To increase the challenge: Set a timer so that you must work against the clock.

Apps for Your Brain

If you'd prefer to use an "app"—a software application that you can use on a smartphone or similar electronic device—there are several good options. Among the best fun/challenging apps (free on Android and Apple)...

•**Words with Friends.** This ever-popular game allows you to play a Scrabble-like game against your friends who have also downloaded the app on an electronic device. The game provides even more benefits if it's used with the time-clock feature.

•**Word Streak with Friends** (formerly Scramble with Friends) is a timed find-a-word game. You can play on your own or with friends.

•**Elevate** was named Apple's Best App of 2014. It provides a structured game environment that feels more like a test, focusing on reading, writing and math skills, than a game. Still, this timed app will give Apple users a good brain challenge.

Tech-free Options

If you'd rather not stare at the screen of a computer or some other electronic device for your brain workout, here are some good options...

•**Tech-free games.** SET is a fast-paced card game that tests your visual perception skills. Players race to find a set of three matching cards (based on color, shape, number or shading) from an array of cards placed on a table.

Bonus: This game can be played by one player or as many people as can fit around the table. The winner of dozens of "Best Game" awards, including the high-IQ group Mensa's Select award, SET is fun for kids and adults alike.

Another good choice: Boggle, which challenges you to create words from a given set of letter cubes within a three-minute period. It can be played by two or more people.

•**Drumming.** Playing any musical instrument requires attention and a keen sense of timing. Basic drumming is a great activity for beginner musicians (especially if you don't have the finger dexterity for piano or guitar).

Even better: Join a drumming circle, which provides the extra challenge of matching your timing and rhythm to the rest of the drummers, along with opportunities for socialization.

Bonus: Research has demonstrated that some forms, such as African djembe drumming, count as a low- to moderate-intensity activity that may reduce blood pressure, which helps protect the brain from blood vessel damage.

•**Meditation.** This practice improves cognitive function and sensory processing and promotes mental focus. Meditating for about 30 minutes daily has also been linked to greater blood flow to the brain and increased gray matter (associated with positive emotions, memory and decision-making). The benefits have even been seen among some people with early-stage neurodegenerative diseases, such as Alzheimer's disease.

A good way to get started: Begin with a simple "mindful eating" exercise—spend the first five minutes of each meal really focusing on what you're eating. Don't talk, read the paper or watch TV…just savor the food. Eventually, you'll want to expand this level of attention to other parts of your day. Such mindfulness habits are a good complement to a regular meditation practice.

•**Coloring.** If you have kids or grandkids, don't just send them off with their crayons. Color with them.

Even better: Get one of the newer breed of coloring books with complex designs for adults. While there hasn't been specific research addressing the brain benefits of coloring, this form of play has been shown to reduce stress in children, and it is thought to boost creativity and have a meditative quality. You can find coloring books made for adults at bookstores and art-supply stores.

Are Brain Games Bogus?

Cynthia R. Green, PhD, clinical psychologist, and founder and president, Memory Arts, LLC, a brain-health and memory fitness consulting service, Montclair, New Jersey. She is also founding director of The Memory Enhancement Program at Mount Sinai School of Medicine in New York City. She is author of *Your Best Brain Ever: A Complete Guide & Workout.* TotalBrainHealth.com

Lumosity makes online brain games. It also made false advertising claims for years, according to the Federal Trade Commission (FTC). "Lumosity preyed on consumers' fears about age-related cognitive decline, suggesting its games could stave off memory loss, dementia and even Alzheimer's disease," according to the FTC. "But Lumosity simply did not have the science to back up its ads." In a settlement, the company agreed to nix the ads and refund $2 million to its one million paying subscribers.

Lumosity's brain games are fun to play, with their addictive inducements to click to test your ability to, for example, match colors or words ever more quickly, and they do sharpen skills such as speed, attention and memory while you play them. But the evidence has been lacking that they lead to real-life changes in how your brain functions in the real world—especially changes that could lead to preventing cognitive decline.

Perhaps what is most shameful, is that the years touting online training as just the "quick fix" that would keep our brains young has masked the real science of what brain fitness is all about, namely engaging in lifestyle behaviors that have been tied to staying sharp.

The Lumosity debacle does not mean that the online brain-training movement is (or should be) dead. Brain games have their place. Games that pit your cognitive skills against the clock do help you hone your attention and memory skills and mental flexibility. Lumosity's games fit into that category—but you can just as easily get them from video games or free apps on your smartphone.

The cognitive science behind brain games continues to evolve, so their potential can't be dismissed. There is promising work in using brain games to prevent, and even treat, depression, for example. A new medical field is emerging that uses neurofeedback—devices that let you see how your brain reacts in real time to your thoughts and emotions—to treat post-traumatic stress disorder (PTSD) and other attention and anxiety disorders.

Someday, new research may well discover that brain games slow down cognitive decline in aging. Or not. Brain games do no harm, and they sharpen certain cognitive skills, so go ahead and play them if you enjoy them. Just don't expect miracles.

In the meantime, it's best to focus on what we know is key to preserving brain health throughout life—regular exercise, a heart-healthy diet, a strong social network and continuing intellectual stimulation. Real brain health science lies in how we live.

How a Harvard Brain Specialist Keeps Her Own Brain Healthy

Marie Pasinski, MD, a memory specialist and neurologist who is on the faculty of Harvard Medical School and a staff neurologist at Massachusetts General Hospital, both in Boston. She is author, with Liz Neporent, of *Chicken Soup for the Soul: Boost Your Brain Power!*

Scientists used to believe that memory and other mental abilities inevitably declined with age. Not anymore. We now know that the brain has the ability to form new neurons and create new neural pathways throughout life. This means that your ability to remember and learn actually can get better as you age.

It doesn't take hard work—or complicated mental "workouts"—to improve mental agility. Here's what Marie Pasinski, MD, a memory specialist at Harvard Medical School, does to keep her own brain healthy...

Hang Out With Friends

Close relationships are good for the brain. We have found that people who have supportive friends (or spouses) and rich social networks have better cognitive function and lower rates of dementia than those who spend more time alone.

When I take a break during my workday to go for a walk, I like to find someone to go with me. Exercising with friends is ideal because you can catch up on one another's lives while you get in shape.

It's not entirely clear why friendships are so important. One reason is purely mental—the brain is stimulated when you share ideas with other people. Mental stimulation increases the number of neurons and the connections among neurons. Social engagement lowers levels of stress hormones, which appear to be toxic to the neurons in the hippocampus—the brain's memory center. It also appears to lower blood pressure and reduce the risk for stroke.

Spend as much time as you can with people you care about—getting together with one close friend can be just as beneficial as hanging out with a group. Meeting new people is beneficial because it adds an extra jolt of stimulation. You can broaden your social network by volunteering or joining community groups.

Don't Live on Autopilot

Routine is seductive. People like going to the same restaurants or taking the same route to work. The problem with routine is that it literally creates mental ruts—the brain uses only preexisting pathways and neural connections to complete familiar tasks. It stops growing and improving.

By embracing new experiences, you stimulate your brain to create neurons and forge additional neural pathways. This happens every time you extend your scope of experience and think in new ways. The more you challenge your brain—even when the "challenge" is as simple as looking at unfamiliar scenery—the more its functions improve.

For me, writing is a new experience. I can't spell to save my life. My worst course in college was English 101. When a friend suggested that I write a book about memory, I immediately dismissed the idea. Then, a few weeks later, I learned that Harvard was offering a course on publishing. I decided to take it. Now I've completed two books.

For me, shifting attention from medicine to writing was a radical change. But any change, even a small one, can help boost memory and thinking. If you take a new route to work, you will see different buildings. You will have to think about where you're going. This alone is enough to stimulate the brain's circuitry.

Work Both Sides of the Brain

A lot of my patients love to do crossword or other puzzles. They enjoy the challenge, and they've heard that mental activities improve memory. They're right—but only up to a point.

The improvements that you get from mental challenges quickly level off as you gain expertise.

Better: In addition to taking on new challenges, do things that work the underused side of your brain. If you're an accountant who crunches numbers all day, you're drawing heavily on the logical left side of the brain. Take up a hobby that works the right side, the imaginative side, such as painting or making pottery.

For me, playing the piano is a creative and welcome distraction from my work in medicine. I tried to learn to play when I was young, but my teacher was awful! I took it up again later in life. This time, I got to choose my own teacher, who has since become a close friend.

Have Fun

People who enjoy what they're doing get a mental boost. "Forcing" yourself to do things that aren't fun won't be anywhere near as good for your brain as activities that you genuinely enjoy. Also, enjoyment triggers the release of dopamine, a neurotransmitter that enhances learning and retention of new material.

I often ask patients to describe some of the things that they would like to do but have never done. Some would like to learn a new language. Others want to take up a new hobby, such as bird-watching or playing a sport. Ideally, whatever you choose will be both unfamiliar and fun.

I've tried all sorts of things in recent years, from joining Facebook and taking improv classes to competing in triathlons and gardening.

Move!

I do something physical every day. I enjoy biking, running, swimming, tennis and skiing. I also take jazz-dance classes.

Exercise triggers the release of brain-derived neurotrophic factor, a growth factor that promotes the formation of new synapses in the brain—the connections among brain cells that are critical for memory and other cognitive functions.

Exercise also increases the size of the brain. In one study, nonexercisers were given MRI scans to measure their brain volume. Then they were instructed to walk for 60 minutes, three days a week. After six months, they were given another MRI. The scans showed that they had an increase in the size of the prefrontal cortex, the part of the brain that is involved in reasoning, problem-solving and other "executive" functions.

Exercise also increases the size of the hippocampus, the area of the brain that is closely involved with memory. It improves circulation and helps prevent hypertension and other conditions that increase the risk for dementia.

Even if you don't enjoy "formal" exercise, you can get similar benefits just by moving more. I spend a lot of time at my computer, but I take a break every hour or so just to move around.

Eat Brain Food

A Mediterranean-style diet, with relatively little red meat and lots of fish, vegetables and whole grains, is the best diet for brain health. People who follow this diet have less atherosclerosis, hypertension and diabetes, conditions that cause inflammation and other brain changes that impair thinking and memory. *Fish and olive oil, two staples of the Mediterranean diet, are particularly good for the brain...*

•**Fish and omega-3s.** About two-thirds of the brain consists of fat. When you eat salmon, sardines or other cold-water fish, the omega-3s from the fish are incorporated into brain tissue. A study published in *American Journal of Clinical Nutrition*, which looked at more than 2,000 men and women ages 70 to 74, found that those who ate, on average, one-third of an ounce or more of fish daily did better on cognitive tests than those who ate less.

I try to eat fish at least a few days a week. If you're not fond of fish, you can get some of the same benefits from eggs or milk that is fortified with omega-3s. Other less potent sources of omega-3s include walnuts, pumpkin seeds and soybeans. You also can take fish-oil supplements. The usual dose is 1,000 milligrams (mg) to 2,000 mg daily. Because the supplements can have a blood-thinning effect and/or interact with some medications, check with your doctor before taking them.

•**Olive oil.** It's a healthy fat that reduces inflammation, improves cholesterol and helps reduce the risk for stroke. I use it for cooking almost every day. People who use olive oil regularly tend to have lower rates of dementia and better cognitive function.

Five Big Brain Myths—Busted!

Sandra Bond Chapman, PhD, a cognitive neuroscientist who is the founder and chief director of the Center for BrainHealth and the Dee Wyly Distinguished University Chair, both at The University of Texas at Dallas. She is coauthor, with Shelly Kirkland, of *Make Your Brain Smarter: Increase Your Brain's Creativity, Energy, and Focus.* Center ForBrainHealth.org

For most people over age 40, glitches in memory are high on their lists of health concerns. Whether it's lost keys, forgotten names or other "senior moments," we fear each is a sign of a deteriorating brain.

What science now tells us: Memory is not necessarily the most important measure of brain health. And no matter what your age, there are ways to improve the mind. However, many of the popular beliefs about improving mental performance are outdated and incorrect.

Most common myths...

MYTH #1: **Brain health steadily declines with age.** Scientists used to believe that people were born with all of the neurons (brain cells) that they'd ever have and that the ability to form new brain connections ended in adolescence.

It's now known that the brain is the most modifiable part of the body. It's constantly being changed by how we use it, and the changes can be measured within just hours. That's why you can be confounded by, say, a new cell phone in the morning and then be using it proficiently by the end of the day.

While you are focused on new learning—such as writing an original report or preparing new recipes—neural activity increases and promotes the development of new neurons. But if these neurons are not put to proper use, they die.

As you age, your ability to think more broadly and deeply can continue to grow if your brain is exercised properly—thanks to the functions of your frontal lobes, the part of your brain that sits just behind and above your eyes in your skull. Even though brain health is tied to all parts of the brain, the majority of the heavy lifting is directed through the frontal lobe networks. The frontal lobes are responsible for decision making, judgment, planning and other "executive" functions.

My advice: Engage your frontal lobes by being curious and creative and by solving problems whenever you can. Challenge your brain by thinking deeply and extracting meaning from information you are given.

Example: Think back to a favorite book that you read several years ago, and come up with five to eight different take-home messages that are applicable to different contexts.

Better yet: Read it again, and then come up with the list.

MYTH #2: **A good memory indicates mental robustness.** Surprisingly, memory skills do not correspond to everyday-life performance as much as frontal lobe functioning. This means that you can have an excellent memory but not be very innovative, insightful, creative or mentally productive.

My advice: Don't worry when you can't remember everything. Although we tend to note what we forget, we rarely take stock of all the things we do remember.

A brain that gets too occupied with remembering everything works less efficiently and becomes stressed, overwhelmed and bogged down in the details. If something is important in your life—it could be your work, a hobby or even a weekly card game—you'll remember the details that really matter.

Do not worry about, say, occasional forgotten names or unimportant tasks. But when forgetting regularly interferes with your performance, it may be a sign that something more than benign memory glitches is taking over. Many things can impair memory—not enough sleep, some medications, such as antidepressants and blood pressure drugs, and stress. Memory issues do not always mean Alzheimer's disease. See your doctor if you're concerned about your memory.

MYTH #3: **Multitasking gives your brain a good workout.** Again, not true. When you multitask, the brain has to call on different regions to handle the load. It works inefficiently because the communication isn't synchronized. When you "overuse" your brain in this way, the frontal lobes become fatigued. This slows efficiency and decreases performance.

My advice: Whatever you're doing, focus on that and nothing else for at least 15 minutes. Put a "do not disturb" sign on the door. Turn off your phones, and don't check your e-mail. You'll think more clearly in those 15 minutes than someone who multitasks for an hour.

MYTH #4: **People with a high IQ have the most brainpower.** Today's IQ tests are based on measurements that were developed more than a century ago. They mainly emphasize such skills as knowledge, memory and speed in ability to perform mathematical equations—all of which were much more important in the days before computers and the Internet.

What's more important is knowing how to use knowledge in novel ways and bringing together facts from disparate areas to create original ideas. As Einstein said, "Imagination is more important than knowledge. Knowledge is limited. Imagination encircles the world."

My advice: Whenever you're confronted with a problem, stop and think deeply about the knowledge you already have. Connecting it and generating original ideas is crucial to brain health.

MYTH #5: **Unrelenting mental work boosts brain capacity.** It's true that high achievers can put in long hours and consider lots of information when

Best Way to Fight Memory Loss

The combination of computer use and exercise is better than mental or physical activity alone. The exact reason is not yet known, but it may be that physical activity improves blood flow to the brain and therefore delivers more nutrients...while mental activity works at the molecular level to boost synaptic activities.

Yonas E. Geda, MD, MSc, a neuropsychiatrist at Mayo Clinic, Scottsdale, Arizona, and leader of a study of 926 people, ages 70 to 93, published in *Mayo Clinic Proceedings*.

they try to solve vexing problems. But they also know when to stop looking at more information—and they reach that point earlier than most people do.

Productivity and achievement are not linked to how many hours are worked and how much information is accessed. In fact, decreasing exposure allows your frontal lobes to be deployed to focus on key data, and, even more importantly, to know what information to ignore.

Using knowledge to support a novel approach is essential to enhancing integrated reasoning and deeper-level thinking.

Example: Instead of taking copious notes on specific points made in a meeting, boil down the discussion to key issues, new decisions and possibilities.

My advice: Keep your key frontal lobe operations finely tuned by blocking, discarding and ignoring less relevant tasks and information. Consolidating facts and options into big ideas and perspectives is necessary to cultivate creative thinking and problem solving.

Are You Shrinking Your Brain?

Daniel G. Amen, MD, a brain-imaging specialist, is the founder, CEO and medical director of the Amen Clinics and author of several books, including *Use Your Brain to Change Your Age: Secrets to Look, Feel, and Think Younger Every Day*.

When scientists talk about memory and learning, the hippocampus, a small, seahorse-shaped structure located deep inside the brain, gets most of the credit for these vital cognitive functions.

What you don't hear much about: The prefrontal cortex (PFC), a much larger part of the brain located just behind and slightly beneath the forehead. Known as the "executive" part of the brain because it controls judgment, insights and impulse control, the PFC is just as important when it comes to staying sharp mentally, learning new information and controlling processes involved in memory.

Unfortunately, millions of Americans don't follow simple lifestyle habits that promote optimal functioning of the PFC.

Result: Lapses in judgment (such as making risky maneuvers when driving)…disorganized thinking (including an inability to prioritize tasks)… shorter attention spans (resulting in difficulty with reading and other activities that require focus)…and impairments in learning and memory.

Improve Your Brain—Live Longer

The PFC needs good "fuel" to thrive. That's why people with healthful habits tend to have a larger PFC than those who don't take good care of themselves. As a result, they're more likely to live longer (because their judgment about risks is better), and they're less likely to develop Alzheimer's disease.

Important finding: A 2007 study of Catholic nuns and priests found that those who had the most self-discipline were 89% less likely to develop Alzheimer's disease. Self-discipline is one of the traits that is enhanced when you have a robust PFC.

Power Up Your "Wiring"

To protect your PFC—and other key parts of the brain…

•**Rethink your alcohol intake.** Millions of Americans drink a glass or two of red wine a day because it's good for the heart. But the cardio-protective properties of alcohol—it raises HDL "good" cholesterol and reduces clots, thus reducing the risk for a heart attack—may be offset by the damage it can do to the brain. Alcohol decreases the size and functioning of the PFC. What's more, even moderate drinking (two drinks daily for men and one for women) can impair brain circulation.

My advice: If your doctor agrees that you can forgo the cardiovascular benefits of drinking wine, limit your intake to no more than two or three alcoholic beverages per week.

•**"Water" your brain.** The brain is 80% water. People who don't drink enough water or who drink a lot of dehydrating liquids, such as alcohol or caffeinated coffee or tea, often have impairments in cognition and judgment, which can occur when the PFC is damaged.

My advice: Drink plenty of water—eight glasses (64 ounces) of water every day is typically sufficient. If you like, add a splash of lemon or lime juice for flavor.

•**Slow down on the omega-6s.** Most Americans get far too many inflammation-promoting omega-6 essential fatty acids in their diets—primarily from cooking oils (such as corn and vegetable), fatty red meats and processed foods—that are harmful to the brain. That's why a plant-based, anti-inflammatory diet is among the most effective ways to reduce damage to the PFC and other areas of the brain.

My advice: Eat lots of greens—including salads—along with vegetables, fruit, whole grains and legumes. Approximately three servings of lean protein daily will help balance blood sugar and keep you feeling sharp. Also, eat at least three servings weekly of cold-water fish such as salmon, mackerel and sardines. The omega-3s in these fish have potent anti-inflammatory effects. Fish oil supplements (1 g to 3 g daily) are also helpful. Check with your doctor first if you use a blood thinner.

Aim to change your diet so that your intake of omega-6 fatty acids is no more than three times higher than your intake of omega-3s.

Good rule of thumb: A plant-based diet that's high in fish provides the ideal 3:1 (or lower) ratio of omega-6s to omega-3s.

•**Try green tea and rhodiola.** Distractibility, disorganization and poor impulse control are commonly associated with children who may be suffering from attention-deficit/hyperactivity disorder (ADHD), but many adults (who may or may not have ADHD) also struggle with such symptoms.

Often linked to low activity in the PFC, these symptoms can be reversed, in part, with green tea and rhodiola, a plant-based supplement frequently used as an energy booster. In one study, researchers at my clinic did brain scans before and after giving patients green tea and rhodiola. Two months later, scans showed a significant increase in circulation in the PFC.

How it helps: Green tea appears to benefit the PFC by increasing the availability of dopamine, a brain chemical that controls the brain's reward and pleasure centers. It also helps regulate emotional responses, such as the motivation to take positive actions. Rhodiola is an "adaptogen," a substance that normalizes the body's functions by boosting blood flow to the brain and raising dopamine and serotonin levels.

My advice: Take 200 mg of rhodiola and drink two to three cups of green tea daily (avoid drinking it in the evening since the tea's caffeine can interfere with sleep…or drink decaffeinated green tea).

•**Keep your BMI in check.** People who are overweight—with a body mass index (BMI) of 25 or higher—have less circulation in the PFC than those of normal weights. Excess body weight is associated with atherosclerosis, diabetes and other conditions that impede circulation throughout the body.

Danger: A high BMI can cause the brain to shrink. Research has shown that people who are obese typically have about 8% less brain tissue than normal-weight adults.

My advice: At least once a year, check your BMI by using an online calculator, such as the National Heart, Lung and Blood Institute's NHLBI.nih.gov/health/educational/lose_wt/bmitools.htm. A BMI of 18.5 to 24.9 is considered normal. If your BMI is 25 or higher, you need to lose weight.

•**Don't ignore sleep problems.** An estimated 18 million Americans have sleep apnea, a condition in which breathing intermittently stops during sleep. Unfortunately, the condition is undiagnosed in most of these people.

Why does this matter? Scans on patients with sleep apnea show brain changes that resemble early Alzheimer's disease. Poor sleep decreases blood flow to the PFC and other parts of the brain. Snoring, daytime fatigue and morning headaches are common symptoms of sleep apnea. Your doctor may recommend tests in a sleep laboratory.

My advice: If you're overweight, sleep apnea can often be reduced or even eliminated with weight loss. Many patients also benefit from continuous positive airway pressure (CPAP) units, which help keep the airways open during sleep.

Also important: Avoid sleepless nights. Patients with chronic insomnia have a higher risk for cognitive declines than people who sleep well. To prevent insomnia, follow the tried-and-true strategies—relax in a warm bath before bed...reduce arousal by not watching TV or using a computer in the hour before bedtime...and go to bed and wake up at the same times every day.

Also helpful: Melatonin. The standard dose of this sleep hormone supplement is 1 mg to 6 mg taken a half hour before bed. Start with the lower dose and increase it over a period of weeks, if necessary.

Check with your doctor first if you take an antidepressant, blood pressure medication, blood thinner, steroid or nonsteroidal anti-inflammatory drug—melatonin may interact with these medications.

Meditate for a Bigger Brain

Eileen Luders, PhD, associate professor, department of neurology, Brain Mapping Center, University of California, Los Angeles, and lead author of a study of 44 people.

Compared with nonmeditators, people who had meditated between 10 and 90 minutes a day for five to 46 years had significantly greater brain volume in some regions linked to emotion, according to brain scans.

Theory: Meditation may promote better nerve connections or larger cells in certain brain regions—which may explain many meditators' emotional stability and mental focus.

Better Brain Regimen for Every Age

Sandra Bond Chapman, PhD, a cognitive neuroscientist, founder and chief director of the Center for BrainHealth and the Dee Wyly Distinguished University Chair at The University of Texas at Dallas. She is coauthor, with Shelly Kirkland, of *Make Your Brain Smarter: Increase Your Brain's Creativity, Energy, and Focus.* BrainHealth.UTDallas.edu

What exactly can you do to improve your mental fitness? Here are some regimens that are geared toward the changes your brain is undergoing as it ages.

AGES 46 TO 65

Beginning in one's mid-40s, it's common to start losing the capacity to quickly process new information and store and retrieve data (such as a person's name). However, most people in the 46-to-65 age group are more adept at sorting through information efficiently and accurately discerning critical points to more quickly weigh facts than younger counterparts.

Best brain-boosting strategies if you're age 46 to 65...

•**Narrow your focus.** Multitasking isn't recommended for anyone, but particularly not for people in this age group. As you age, the capacity to rapidly switch from task to task (as occurs with multitasking) slows, adding to brain fatigue and reducing efficiency.

To keep the mind sharp: Pick one job—such as answering e-mails or planning a report—and take your time doing it. Making an effort to create meaningful responses and original content not only increases work quality and productivity but also flexes your brain.

•**Synthesize.** Not every detail is important, so don't let yourself get lost in a sea of information.

To keep the mind sharp: Gather enough information for the task at hand, then focus mainly on the key meanings. Applying internally generated novel ideas to affect an outcome boosts brain health.

Note: Don't feel insecure because your grasp of details may not be what it used to be. This can be a strength—it means that you're more likely to see the bigger picture.

AGES 66 AND OLDER

You may notice increasing incidences of memory glitches, but it is probably not as dramatic as you think. People tend to notice when they forget a few minor details, such as the name of the movie they saw last month. They don't consider the tens of thousands of details that they didn't forget.*

Try to nourish your brain by putting accumulated knowledge and wisdom to work. Deep thinking and disciplined use of brainpower helps fine-tune brain resources for optimal performance.

Best brain-boosting strategies if you're age 66 or older...

•**Get off autopilot.** At this age, you are especially at risk for slipping into autopilot—a dangerous state, since a bored brain is going backward.

To keep the mind sharp: Continue to push yourself to learn something new, especially if it's related to technology, which can help build new connections in the brain. You will feel energized as you go from being a novice to an expert in an area of interest.

•**Stay challenged.** The problem with crossword puzzles and other brain teasers is that they get easier with practice. People who do crosswords get better mainly at crosswords, and the gains generally don't translate into other high-level mental areas.

To keep the mind sharp: Take on real challenges that you are motivated to master. Forcing yourself to learn a new language just to exercise your brain will not produce the same far-reaching cognitive benefits as honing a foreign language for practical use, such as for a trip. The brain expands and develops new pathways when it's pushed to explore unfamiliar areas.

*If problems with memory or decision-making begin to interfere with daily life, such as completing household tasks, consult your doctor.

Fortifying Younger Brains

Adults who are under age 45 tend to be very comfortable with collecting facts—but they often are less confident than they could be when dealing with abstract concepts and making decisions. *How people in this age group can improve their brain performance…*

•**Don't get distracted.** Younger adults have a tremendous ability to memorize, but they're typically poor at choosing what they need to remember. Most people will function just fine if they ignore about 50% of the information that comes their way.

Helpful: Focus on accomplishing your top two or three priorities for the day without letting distractions, such as constant text, e-mail and social-media alerts, disrupt your progress.

•**Zoom out.** When every fact in the world is a click away, our brains often get stuck regurgitating facts and blindly following directions.

Helpful: When you're reading for knowledge (not for entertainment), skim the material quickly…find the takeaway message…and then condense it to a succinct thought. Translating new information into your own words increases comprehension and helps you achieve new perspectives that can inspire your brain to generate new ideas and solutions.

Surprising Brain Booster

Paul Nussbaum, PhD, clinical neuropsychologist and president of the Brain Health Center, Wexford, Pennsylvania. PaulNussbaum.com

Some people love to travel. But if you're someone who needs a good reason to pack your bags, here's one to consider: Your brain will love it if you hit the road!

Here's why: The brain's ability to grow, known as plasticity, never stops. When you take in new sights and information—walking unfamiliar streets, admiring the scenery and listening to (and speaking) unfamiliar languages—the brain forms new neurons and connections. It literally gets bigger and more vibrant.

You may also get a boost in creativity. Research that looked at fashion executives found that those who had lived abroad created products that were consistently more creative than those produced by their stay-at-home peers.

Of course, not everyone has the time (or the cash or inclination) for exotic vacations. That's OK. Your brain will also be happy with a stimulating "staycation."

The trick: Do anything that isn't routine. Go on weekend road trips. Visit that museum you've always been meaning to see. Introduce yourself to someone whom you've been tempted to talk to but never did.

But if you can travel, go ahead and book those tickets. Even when the trip is over, you'll hopefully have photos to remind you of your adventures and memories to share with others. Remembering stimulates the same neurochemistry as the experience itself. Your brain wants to be stimulated, and reliving your travels is yet another great way to do it.

How Google Exercises Your Brain

Gary Small, MD, director of the Longevity Center at the Semel Institute for Neuroscience & Human Behavior, University of California, Los Angeles. He is also coauthor of many books, including *iBrain, Snap! Change Your Personality in 30 Days* and *2 Weeks to a Younger Brain.* DrGarySmall.com

Can you use the Internet to better your brain? Yes, say researchers at University of California at Los Angeles who conducted a study called "Your Brain on Google." The research team, led by Gary Small, MD, of UCLA's Longevity Center, explored whether searching the Internet stimulates areas of the brain that control decision making, complex reasoning and vision. The researchers discovered it does, but only for those who use Google or other search engines in a certain way.

Net-Net...

The study included 24 people aged 55 to 76. Half the subjects (the "Net Naïve" group) had little or no experience in searching the Internet, while the other half (the "Net Savvy" group) were skilled computer users who regularly use the Internet. This age group was chosen because researchers postulated that age-related brain changes are associated with declines in cognitive abilities, such as processing speed and working memory, and that routine computer use might

Better Brain-Building Activities

Retired adults age 75 and older who held demanding jobs that required strategic thinking, verbal skills and some advanced-level education scored higher on cognitive tests over an eight-year period than adults whose jobs did not.

Explanation: These skills use areas of the brain that build a cognitive reserve, which helps protect memory and thinking abilities.

Even if you didn't have this type of job, you can still develop cognitive skills after retirement by doing volunteer work that involves organization and planning.

Francisca S. Then, PhD, research fellow, Institute for Social Medicine, Occupational Health and Public Health, University of Leipzig, Germany.

have an impact—negative or positive. Both groups were asked to perform two tasks. First, to read text on a computer screen, and second to use Google to search the web. The reading material and research topics were interesting and similar in content (for instance, the benefits of drinking coffee, planning a trip to the Galapagos Islands, how to choose a car, etc.).

Meanwhile, as the subjects worked on their computers, researchers scanned their brains with a functional magnetic resonance imaging (fMRI) device to ascertain which parts were active. During the text-reading phase, these fMRI scans revealed similar activity for both groups in the regions that control language, reading, memory and vision.

But there were very dissimilar results when the two groups performed Web searches. When the Net Naïve group searched the Internet, their brain activity was similar to what they had experienced while reading…in contrast, the Net Savvy group produced activity in areas of the brain that control decision making and complex reasoning. Previous studies have shown that this type of brain activity is important for everyday cognitive tasks.

Engaging Content

This result shows that the Internet is itself "brain stimulation." This may be especially helpful as people age because, compared with reading, Web searches require making more decisions. For instance, searchers must decide which information to pursue and which to ignore. The Net Naïve group may show less brain stimulation than the Net Savvy group because of their inexperience with the Internet. When this group was given some training their brains showed similar patterns of activity to those who were adept at Internet use.

So, if you haven't been very involved with using your computer to research topics of interest, give it a try—it's great mental exercise.

Learn a Word a Day and Other Fun Ways to Add Healthy Years to Your Life

The late **Robert N. Butler, MD,** former president and chief executive officer of the International Longevity Center-USA. He also was professor of geriatrics at Brookdale Department of Geriatrics and Adult Development at Mount Sinai Medical Center in New York City. He wrote *The Longevity Prescription: The 8 Proven Keys to a Long, Healthy Life* and won the 1976 Pulitzer Prize for his book *Why Survive? Being Old in America.*

We all know that eating right and exercising can boost our chances of a long, healthy life. But sometimes it seems as if the changes we have to make to live a healthier life are simply too overwhelming. The good news is that just a few little changes can have a significant impact on our health. *Here, the little changes that can make a big difference…*

●**Learn a word a day.** Pick a word out of the paper or dictionary every day. Or have a word e-mailed to you daily (Dictionary.Reference.com/wordofthe-day). Put it on an index card, and drill yourself. This type of cognitive calisthenic keeps your brain sharp.

The brain continues to regenerate nerve cells throughout life. This process, known as neurogenesis, helps older adults to improve memory and other cognitive functions as they age.

Example: A 2006 study published in *The Journal of the American Medical Association* compared two groups of older adults. Those in one group were given training in memory, reasoning and mental processing. After just 10 sessions of 60 to 75 minutes each, the participants had immediate and long-lasting improvements, compared with those who didn't get the training.

> ### Fight Dementia By Learning a Second Language
>
> In a study of people with dementia, bilingual people developed dementia about five years later than people who spoke just one language.
>
> *Possible reason:* Switching from one language to another in the course of routine communication helps to stimulate the brain.
>
> Study of the medical records of 648 people, average age 66, by researchers at University of Edinburgh, Scotland, and Nizam's Institute of Medical Sciences, Hyderabad, India, published in *Neurology.*

If learning a word a day doesn't appeal to you, pick an activity that you enjoy and find mentally challenging.

Examples: Reading history books, learning chess or memorizing poems. When the activity starts getting easier, move on to harder challenges.

People who do this can regain as much as two decades of memory power. In other words, someone who starts at age 70 could achieve the memory of the average 50-year-old.

•**Make social connections.** Go on a cruise. Take a bus tour. Go to a reunion. All of these are great ways to connect with people. Why bother? Because emotional connections add years to your life.

Example: Studies published in the last 10 years show that people in happy marriages have less heart disease and live longer than those in unhappy relationships or who are divorced or widowed. Being happily married at age 50 is a better predictor of good health at age 80 than having low cholesterol.

The same benefits occur when people maintain any close relationship—with friends, children or even pets. People who are emotionally bonded with others suffer less depression. They also tend to have less stress and lower levels of disease-causing stress hormones. And inviting new people into your life can help you cope with the dislocations—due to death, divorce, retirement, etc.—that occur over time.

Emotional connections don't just happen—people have to work at them. Think of the friendships that are important to you. If you are like most people, maybe a few of these relationships are active, but others have gone dormant for a variety of reasons. Ask yourself why some relationships have lapsed and what you can do to revive them. If you have lost touch with someone special, send an e-mail or pick up the phone.

We all have "relationship opportunities" that we can take advantage of. Talk to the stranger next to you at a concert or a sports event. If you volunteer, invite one of your coworkers for coffee.

•**Take a nap.** It's a myth that older people need less sleep than younger adults. They often do sleep less, but this is mainly because they're more likely to have physical issues, such as arthritis or the need to use the bathroom at night, that interfere with restful sleep.

People who don't get enough sleep often have declines in immune function, which can increase the risk for cancer as well as infections. They also have a higher risk for hypertension and possibly prediabetes.

A short nap—no more than 20 to 30 minutes—can make up for a bad night's sleep. But beware of excessive napping. A long nap or more than one short nap per day can ruin a good night's sleep. Napping late in the day, say, after 3:00, also can interfere with a night's sleep.

•**Climb the stairs.** It takes very little time but is a great way to get your heart and lungs working. Most exercise guidelines recommend at least 20 to 30 minutes of exercise most days of the week. That much exercise, or more, is clearly beneficial, but short amounts of activity can have a significant impact.

In a study of 5,000 people over age 70, all the participants had some physical limitations, but those who got even minimal exercise (defined as the equivalent of walking a mile at least once a week) were 55% less likely to develop more serious physical limitations (defined as severe joint pain or muscle weakness) that could compromise independence.

●**Watch the birds.** For many people, contact with the natural world has a restorative effect. A few minutes observing birds at a feeder or watching a sunset can restore our equilibrium. The natural world has a pace that reminds us that life does not have to be lived in a rush.

Taking a few moments to destress is worth doing because an estimated 60% of all doctor visits are for stress-related disorders.

Connecting with nature also can boost our performance. A study at Kansas State University gave 90 women a five-minute typing assignment. The researchers found that those who worked with a bouquet of flowers nearby outperformed those with no flowers.

●**See a funny movie.** A good guffaw is more complicated than most people imagine. Laughter involves 15 facial muscles, along with the lungs, larynx and epiglottis. It even seems to protect against heart disease.

A study at Loma Linda University School of Medicine found that volunteers who watched a humorous video had reduced levels of the stress hormones cortisol and epinephrine. These and other stress-related chemicals have been linked with increased inflammation and an elevated risk for heart disease and many other conditions.

The Ultimate Brainpower Workout: If You Exercise the Right Way, You Can Reduce Your Risk for Alzheimer's by Up to 50%

John J. Ratey, MD, an associate clinical professor of psychiatry at Harvard Medical School and a psychiatrist at the Beth Israel-Deaconess Massachusetts Mental Health Center, both in Boston. An adjunct professor at the National Taiwan Sports University, he is author, with Eric Hagerman, of *Spark: The Revolutionary New Science of Exercise and the Brain.* JohnRatey.com

We have known for a long time that exercise helps keep our bodies fit. *Now:* More and more evidence shows that exercise also promotes brain fitness. For example, a study recently published in *Archives of*

Neurology showed that moderate-intensity exercise reduced the odds of developing mild cognitive impairment, which often precedes Alzheimer's disease, by 30% to 40% in the 1,324 study participants (median age 80).

But what type of exercise does the best job of strengthening the brain, and how much is needed for optimal effect?

What you need to know...

The Aging Brain

After age 40, we lose about 5% of our brain cells (neurons) per decade—a process that often accelerates in those who are age 70 and older.

Since the average person has hundreds of billions of neurons, his/her cognitive reserves—that is, the brain's healthy cells that help compensate for damage by recruiting other brain areas to assist with tasks—may be sufficient to maintain mental agility...but not always.

The risk: Millions of Americans who are middle-aged and older start to "slip" in their mental capacities. Even if they have no signs of dementia, it may be harder for them to remember words, names or people than it once was. Or they may struggle to learn new information or take longer to think through problems and find solutions.

Why does this gradual mental decline affect some people much more than others?

Age-related loss of neurons, which affects all of us as we grow older, is just one factor. There's also a decline in dopamine, a neurotransmitter that controls motivation and motor function. This decline interferes with the electrical signals in the brain that allow the remaining neurons to communicate, which is necessary for memory, speech and other key brain functions.

Stronger Body, Bigger Brain

Scientists now know that the brain has plasticity, the ability to form new neurons and connections between neurons. This process can increase the brain's ability to take in information, process it and remember it.

What few people realize: Researchers have now identified a molecule—brain-derived neurotrophic factor (BDNF)—that's largely responsible for plasticity, and its levels increase dramatically with exercise. In animal studies at the University of California, Irvine, mice that exercised regularly were found to have BDNF levels that were about four times higher than those in sedentary mice. Many researchers think that humans show a similar increase.

The BDNF molecule could explain, in part, why people who exercise tend to have less memory loss, are less prone to anxiety and depression, and have up to a 50% lower risk of developing Alzheimer's disease or other forms of dementia than those who are sedentary.

Best exercises for the brain...

The Aerobic Formula

For overall fitness, the Centers for Disease Control and Prevention recommends doing some form of aerobic exercise, such as walking, for 30 minutes at least five days a week. But that's not enough for brain fitness.

Walking at an easy pace might increase your heart rate to about 50% of its maximum. But this has little effect on the brain. For optimal brain benefits, you need to exercise hard enough so that your heart is pumping at 70% to 75% of its maximum rate.* Many treadmills have built-in heart-rate monitors, and heart-rate monitors that you wear are available at most pharmacies.

Good brands of heart-rate monitors: Garmin, Polar and Timex.

Important finding: One study published in *Archives of Neurology* found that people who walked or jogged on a treadmill for 35 minutes at a moderate intensity had improvements in cognitive flexibility (the ability to think flexibly and creatively, rather than merely repeating information) after just one session.

My advice: Exercise at a moderate intensity for 45 minutes to an hour, six days a week.

Remember, a moderate-intensity aerobic workout means elevating your heart rate to 70% to 75% of its maximum capacity. At this rate, you will most likely break a sweat and/or have difficulty carrying on a conversation. You can achieve this by jogging, bicycling, swimming or walking briskly—and then pushing yourself harder when the exercise starts to feel easy.

Example: Once you're comfortable walking for 45 minutes to an hour at the pace described above, increase the intensity by walking faster, swinging your arms or holding hand weights.

If a moderate intensity is too much for you, exercising at 60% of your maximum heart rate has also been shown to offer some improvement in cognitive health.

*To calculate your maximum heart rate, subtract your age from 220. The goal is to exercise at an intensity that raises your pulse to 70% to 75% of your maximum heart rate. The average 65-year-old man, for example, will need to raise his heart rate to about 108 to 116 beats per minute.

Cross Training

To add variety to your aerobic exercise regimen, try some form of cross training. It combines different forms of exercise to target various parts of the body. Circuit training, in which you move quickly from one exercise machine to the next without pausing, is one form of cross training. Another is swimming followed by fast walking.

Cross training is useful because it generally results in a prolonged elevation in heart rate, the critical factor for generating BDNF. Cross training is desirable because it challenges not only your aerobic capacity and strength but also calls upon parts of the brain that govern coordination, planning, etc.

My advice: Whenever possible, incorporate some form of cross training into your regular workouts. In addition, balance exercises are a good way to round out your regimen. Try to work balance exercises, such as tai chi or even any fast-paced form of dancing, into your schedule once or twice a week. These exercises are especially good because they increase your heart rate and require you to think about what you're doing.

Bonus: The social interaction that occurs in tai chi or dance classes and other group activities increases serotonin, a neurotransmitter that reduces anxiety and depression, both of which can impair cognitive functions.

The Power of Mood Workouts

Research shows that the hippocampus (the brain's memory center) is 15% smaller in depressed individuals than in those without depression. Exercise may be one of the most effective ways to reverse depression—perhaps because it influences the same neurochemicals that are affected by antidepressants.

My advice: If you suffer from depression, be sure to follow the exercise guidelines described above. This may allow you to reduce or even eliminate antidepressant medication.

Don't Forget Mental Workouts

Many different studies have shown that higher levels of education are associated with a decreased risk for dementia. But it doesn't matter where you went to school—or even if you went to school. The key factor is continued learning.

Like physical activity, mental workouts increase the number of connections between neurons that enhance memory and cognitive functions.

Perform mental workouts as often as possible.

Good choices: Try vocabulary quizzes, read books on subject matters you're not already familiar with or do any activity that requires you to push yourself intellectually.

Yoga Improves Brain Power More Than Aerobic Exercise

Edward McAuley, PhD, professor, University of Illinois at Urbana-Champaign, Urbana, Illinois. This study was published in *Journal of Physical Activity & Health.*

A good workout can help your brain as much as your body, you've no doubt heard. That's one reason why so many people go for a run when they want to clear their heads. But did you know that, when it comes to boosting your mental prowess, you're probably better off striking a yoga pose than hitting the track or treadmill? *A recent study shows why…*

Participants included 30 adults who did not regularly practice yoga or any similar type of mind-body based exercise (such as tai chi). Each came to the study center on three separate days and took tests designed to measure various aspects of cognitive function.

On one day, they did no exercise prior to taking the tests. On another day, they did 20 minutes of yoga poses, focusing on their breathing and ending with a brief seated meditation, then immediately took the cognitive tests. And on yet another day, they ran on a treadmill for 20 minutes (getting their heart rates up to 60% to 70% of maximum) and then took the same cognitive tests.

The results were surprising—because the participants scored significantly higher after doing yoga than after an aerobic workout or after no exercise. *Specifically…*

•**One test measured inhibitory control, the ability to ignore irrelevant information and maintain focus on relevant items.** On a computer screen, the participants saw numerous rows of arrows facing left or right and had to press the arrow on the keyboard that corresponded to the direction of the arrows in a certain "target" position.

Results: The average score for correct responses after yoga was 90%…but just 83% after running, which was about the same as after no exercise.

•**Another test looked at working memory** (which is responsible for creating and storing memories and retrieving information), with the participants having to remember ever-changing sequences of shapes and respond as quickly as possible.

Results: The average score was 87% after yoga…but just 77% after running and 78% after no exercise. Response time also was faster after yoga—an average of 0.55 seconds, compared with 0.64 seconds after running and 0.60 seconds after no exercise.

Explanation: The researchers offered several possible reasons why yoga boosts brain power. Other studies have shown that yoga improves mood, and better mood is associated with better cognitive function. Yoga also reduces the anxiety that can get in the way of tasks that require full attention. In addition, yoga's emphasis on body awareness and breath control may help enhance the ability to concentrate.

Some questions remain, of course. This study did not demonstrate how long the mental performance-enhancing benefits of yoga might last, given that the participants took their cognitive tests within five minutes after finishing their yoga sessions. And the participants in this study were all women, so we can't say for sure whether men would benefit similarly (though it makes sense that they would).

Still, provided you have your doctor's go-ahead to do yoga, there's certainly no harm—and potentially much to be gained—in doing some yoga poses whenever you feel in need of a brain boost or are about to tackle some challenging mental task.

For inspiration and pose illustrations: Check out the *Yoga Journal* website, YogaJournal.com

CHAPTER 7

Brain Foods and Supplements

The Groundbreaking Alzheimer's Prevention Diet

Richard S. Isaacson, MD, director of the Alzheimer's Prevention Clinic, Weill Cornell Memory Disorders Program at Weill Cornell Medicine and NewYork-Presbyterian, New York City. He is coauthor of *The Alzheimer's Prevention & Treatment Diet: Using Nutrition to Combat the Effects of Alzheimer's Disease.*

As head of the renowned Alzheimer's Prevention Clinic at Weill Cornell Medicine and NewYork-Presbyterian, Richard S. Isaacson, MD, is on top of the latest research on Alzheimer's disease. Groundbreaking studies show that proper diet can make a real difference not only in slowing the progression of the disease but also in preventing it.

Here, Dr. Isaacson explains how we can change our eating habits to fight Alzheimer's. His recommendations are not specifically designed for weight loss, but most overweight people who follow this eating plan will lose weight—important because obesity more than triples the risk for Alzheimer's.

Fewer Calories

The Okinawa Centenarian Study (an ongoing study of centenarians in the Japanese prefecture of Okinawa) found that these long-lived people typically consume fewer calories (up to 1,900 calories a day) than the average American (up to 2,600 calories).

Lowering calorie intake appears to reduce beta-amyloid, particles of protein that form brain plaques—the hallmark of Alzheimer's disease. A 2012 study at the Mayo Clinic found that people who overate had twice the risk for memory loss...and those who consumed more than 2,142 calories a day were more likely to have cognitive impairment.

I generally advise my patients to try to have fewer than 2,100 calories a day. I can't give an exact number because calorie requirements depend on body type, activity level, etc. Many of my patients tend to consume less than 1,800 calories a day, which may be even more protective.

Bonus: Calorie restriction also lowers insulin, body fat, inflammation and blood pressure, all of which can reduce the risk for cognitive impairment. It even improves neurogenesis, the formation of new brain cells.

Less Carbs, More Ketones

Glucose from the breakdown of carbohydrates is the fuel that keeps the body running. But you don't need a lot of carbs. Ketones, another source of fuel, are healthier for the brain.

When you restrict carbohydrates, the body manufactures ketones from stored fat. On occasion, a "ketogenic diet" is recommended for some patients with Alzheimer's disease because ketones produce fewer wastes and put less stress on damaged brain cells. There's some evidence that this diet improves mild cognitive impairment symptoms (and theoretically may slow further damage).

We previously found in our clinic that patients consumed an average of 278 grams of carbohydrates daily before their first visits. We recommend reducing that slowly over the nine weeks of the diet plan to 100 to 120 grams of carbohydrates daily. (One sweet potato has about 23 grams.) Eat healthful carbohydrates such as beans and whole grains in moderation. Unlike refined carbs, they are high in fiber and can help to reduce insulin resistance and improve blood sugar control—which reduces risk for Alzheimer's.

Fasting

Some trendy diets recommend extreme fasts. With the Alzheimer's prevention diet, you'll fast—but mainly when you wouldn't be eating anyway, during sleep!

Several times a week, you'll go without food (particularly carbohydrates) for more than 12 hours. After 12 hours, the body starts making ketones. This type of fast, known as time-restricted eating, reduces inflammation, improves metabolic efficiency and improves insulin levels, insulin sensitivity and brain health.

How to do it: Eat an early supper—say, at about 5 pm. You won't eat again until after 5 am the next day. Your eventual goal will be to fast for 12 to 14 hours five nights a week.

More Protein

The Institute of Medicine recommends getting 10% to 35% of calories from protein—go for the higher end. On a 2,000-calorie diet, that's about 175 grams. (Five ounces of cooked salmon has about 36 grams of protein.)

The amino acids in protein are important for memory and other brain functions. Protein-rich foods often are high in B vitamins, including folic acid and vitamins B-6 and B-12. The Bs are critical because they reduce homocysteine, an amino acid linked to poor brain performance and an increased Alzheimer's risk.

Which protein: Chicken, fish, nuts, legumes and eggs all are good choices. I recommend limiting red meat to one weekly serving because of potential associated health risks, including an increased risk for certain cancers…and because too much saturated fat (see below) can be a problem.

Helpful: Aim for four to eight eggs a week. They're high in selenium, lutein, zeaxanthin and other brain-healthy antioxidants.

Limit Saturated Fat

A large study found that people who eat a lot of foods high in saturated fat—rich desserts, red meat, fast food, etc.—may be up to 2.4 times more likely to develop Alzheimer's disease.

Saturated fat limits the body's ability to "clear" beta-amyloid deposits from the brain. It also raises cholesterol and increases the risk for cardiovascular diseases—and what's bad for the heart also is bad for the brain.

Consuming some saturated fat is healthful—it's only in excess that it causes problems. The American Heart Association advises limiting it to about 5% to 6% of total calories. I recommend a little more—up to 10% of your daily calories. On a 2,000-calorie diet, the upper limit would be about 20 grams. (One ounce of cheese can have as much as eight grams.)

Fish, Turmeric and Cocoa

Studies have shown that a few specific foods can fight Alzheimer's...

•**Fish.** A UCLA study found that adults who regularly ate foods high in omega-3 fatty acids (the healthful fats in fish) had a lower risk for mental decline. Other research has shown that low blood levels of DHA (a type of omega-3) are linked to smaller brain volume and lower scores on cognitive tests.

My advice: Eat one serving of fatty fish (such as wild salmon, mackerel and sardines) at least twice a week. (For more on fish and the brain, see the next two articles.)

•**Turmeric.** In India, where people use the spice turmeric frequently, the risk for Alzheimer's is lower than in the US. This doesn't prove that turmeric is responsible (genetic factors, for example, also could be involved), but other evidence suggests that it's protective. Turmeric contains the compound curcumin, which has potent antioxidant and anti-inflammatory effects.

My advice: Use the spice in recipes—don't depend on supplements—because curcumin is fat-soluble and absorption is enhanced by the fat in foods.

•**Cocoa.** The flavanols in cocoa improve memory and other cognitive functions. They also have been linked to reduced blood pressure and improved insulin resistance.

My advice: Buy chocolate bars or cocoa powder that list purified cocoa flavanols on the label.

The Diet That Cuts Your Alzheimer's Risk in Half

Martha Clare Morris, ScD, professor and director of the Section of Nutrition and Nutritional Epidemiology at Rush University, Chicago, where she is assistant provost for community research. She specializes in dietary and other preventable risk factors in the development of Alzheimer's disease and other chronic diseases in older adults.

Some of the same diets that are good for cardiovascular health also are good for the brain. But there's a new diet—combining the best aspects of other diets—that is so effective it reduces the risk for Alzheimer's disease even in those who don't give the diet their best effort.

The MIND diet blends components from DASH (a blood pressure–lowering diet) and the popular Mediterranean diet, with an extra emphasis on berries, leafy greens and a few other brain-healthy foods.

How good is it? People who carefully followed the diet were about 53% less likely to develop Alzheimer's disease in subsequent years. Those who approached it more casually didn't do quite as well but still reduced their risk considerably, by about 35%.

Blended Benefits

The MIND diet was developed by researchers at Rush University who examined years of studies to identify specific foods and nutrients that seemed to be particularly good—or bad—for long-term brain health. The MIND (it stands for Mediterranean-DASH Intervention for Neurodegenerative Delay) diet is a hybrid plan that incorporates the "best of the best."

In a study in the journal *Alzheimer's & Dementia*, the researchers followed more than 900 participants. None had dementia when the study started. The participants filled out food questionnaires and had repeated neurological tests over a period averaging more than four years.

Some participants followed the MIND diet. Others followed the older DASH diet or the Mediterranean diet. All three diets reduced the risk for Alzheimer's disease. But only the MIND diet did so even when the participants followed the plan only "moderately well."

This is an important distinction because few people are perfect about sticking to diets. Most cheat now and then and eat more unhealthy foods than they should.

The MIND diet specifies "brain-healthy" food groups and five groups that need to be limited, either eaten in moderation or preferably not at all.

What to Eat

•**More leafy greens.** Kale really is a superfood for the brain. So are spinach, chard, beet greens and other dark, leafy greens. The Mediterranean and DASH diets advise people to eat more vegetables, but they don't specify which ones.

The MIND diet specifically recommends one serving of greens a day, in addition to one other vegetable. Previous research has shown that a vegetable-rich diet can help prevent cognitive decline, but two of the larger studies found that leafy greens were singularly protective.

•**Lots of nuts.** The diet calls for eating nuts five times a week. Nuts are high in vitamin E and monounsaturated and polyunsaturated fats—all good for brain health.

The study didn't look at which nuts were more likely to be beneficial. Eating a variety is probably a good idea because you'll get a varied mix of protective nutrients and antioxidants. Raw or roasted nuts are fine (as long as they're not roasted in fat and highly salted). If you are allergic to nuts, seeds such as sunflower and pumpkin seeds are good sources of these nutrients as well.

•**Berries.** These are the only fruits that are specifically included in the MIND diet. Other fruits are undoubtedly good for you, but none has been shown in studies to promote cognitive health. Berries, on the other hand, have been shown to slow age-related cognitive decline. In laboratory studies, a berry-rich diet improves memory and protects against abnormal changes in the brain. Blueberries seem to be particularly potent. Eat berries at least twice a week.

•**Beans and whole grains.** These fiber-rich and folate-rich foods provide high levels of protein with much less saturated fat than you would get from an equivalent helping of meat. The MIND diet calls for three daily servings of whole grains and three weekly servings of beans.

•**Include fish and poultry—but you don't need to go overboard.** Seafood is a key component of the Mediterranean diet, and some proponents recommend eating it four times a week or more. The MIND diet calls for only one weekly serving, although more is OK. A once-a-week fish meal is enough for brain health.

There is no data to specify the number of poultry servings needed for brain health, but we recommend two servings a week.

•**A glass of wine.** People who drink no wine—or those who drink too much—are more likely to suffer cognitive declines than those who drink just a little.

Recommended: One glass a day. Red wine, in particular, is high in flavonoids and polyphenols that may be protective for the brain.

Foods to Limit

•**Limit red meat, cheese, butter and margarine**—along with fast food, fried food and pastries and other sweets. The usual suspects, in other words.

All of these food groups increase the risk for Alzheimer's disease, probably because of their high levels of saturated fat (or, in the case of some margarines, trans fats). Saturated fat has been linked to higher cholesterol, more systemic inflammation and possibly a disruption of the blood-brain barrier that may allow harmful substances into the brain.

However, most nutritionists acknowlege the importance of letting people enjoy some treats and not being so restrictive that they give up eating healthfully altogether.

Try to follow these recommendations...

Red meat: No more than three servings a week.

Butter and margarine: Less than one tablespoon daily. Cook with olive oil instead.

Cheese: Less than one serving a week.

Pastries and sweets: Yes, you can enjoy some treats, but limit yourself to five servings or fewer a week.

Fried or fast food: Less than one serving a week.

Brain Food for the Sexes

Daniel G. Amen, MD, a brain-imaging specialist and medical director of Amen Clinics. Based in Newport Beach, California, he is author of numerous books, including *Unleash the Power of the Female Brain.* AmenClinics.com

Women and men need different foods. The reason? They have very different brains.

We did a study of 46,000 brain scans involving about 26,000 patients. Using a brain-imaging test called SPECT (single photon emission computed tomography), we found clear differences between male and female brains.

In general: Women's brains are more active than men's brains. Much of this activity is in the region known as the prefrontal cortex, which controls judgment, impulse control and organization. Women also produce less serotonin than men. Serotonin is the neurotransmitter that makes you less worried and more relaxed, so women are more prone to anxiety and depression.

Men, on the other hand, produce less dopamine. Dopamine is involved with focus and impulse control, so men are more likely to be impulsive and have trouble concentrating.

Best Foods for Women

Foods that increase serotonin are critical for women. When their serotonin levels rise, women naturally experience less anxiety and are less likely to get upset...

•**Chickpeas.** Also known as garbanzo beans, chickpeas increase the brain's production of serotonin. Other carbohydrates do the same thing, but chickpeas are better because they're high in nutrients and fiber, with about 12 grams of fiber per one-cup serving. Fiber slows the body's absorption of sugars… prevents sharp spikes in insulin…and helps the brain work at optimal levels.

•**Sweet potatoes.** They're my favorite starch because they taste good, are high in vitamin C and fiber and don't raise blood sugar/insulin as quickly as white potatoes. They're a "smart" carbohydrate that causes a gradual increase in serotonin.

•**Blueberries.** They're called "brain berries" for a reason. Blueberries are a concentrated source of flavonoids and other antioxidants that reduce brain inflammation. This is important for good mood and memory. Studies have shown that people who eat blueberries may have less risk for dementia-related cognitive declines.

You will get some of the same benefits with other berries, including strawberries, but blueberries are a better choice for brain function.

•**Dark chocolate.** It is one of the healthiest foods that you can eat. Chocolate increases levels of nitric oxide, a molecule that dilates arteries throughout the body, including those in the brain. One study found that women who ate the most chocolate had greater improvements in verbal fluency and other mental functions than those who ate the least. Chocolate also can improve your mood and energy levels. Because it's high in antioxidants, it reduces the "oxidative stress" that can impair memory and other brain functions. I recommend dark chocolate with natural sweeteners.

Best Foods for Men

Men naturally gravitate to high-protein foods. The protein increases dopamine and provides fuel for a man's greater muscle mass. The trick for men is choosing healthier protein sources…

•**Salmon.** Between 15% and 20% of the brain's cerebral cortex consists of docosahexaenoic acid (DHA), one of the omega-3 fatty acids found in salmon and other fatty fish such as tuna, trout, sardines, herring and mackerel. Men who don't eat fish are more likely to have brain inflammation that can impair the transmission of nerve signals.

A study published in *Alzheimer's & Dementia: The Journal of the Alzheimer's Association* found that elderly adults who got more DHA had improvements in memory and learning. The study focused on supplements, but you can get plenty of DHA and other omega-3s by eating fatty fish more often.

• **Eggs.** They are not the dietary danger that people once thought. Recent research has shown that people who eat a few eggs a week—or even as many as one a day—are no more likely to develop heart disease or have a stroke than those who don't eat eggs.

Eggs are an excellent source of protein, inexpensive and easy to prepare. They also are high in vitamin B-12, which can reduce age-related brain shrinkage and improve cognitive function.

• **Sesame seeds and Brazil nuts.** In addition to increasing dopamine, they contain antioxidants that protect brain cells. Like other nuts and seeds, they're high in protein and monounsaturated fats that reduce LDL "bad" cholesterol.

Nuts and seeds are good for the heart as well as the brain. The landmark Adventist Health Study, conducted by researchers at Loma Linda University, found that people who ate nuts five or more times a week were only about half as likely to have a heart attack as those who rarely ate them.

For a Sharper Brain, Eat These Four Foods

Drew Ramsey, MD, an assistant clinical professor of psychiatry at Columbia University College of Physicians and Surgeons in New York City. Dr. Ramsey is also coauthor of *The Happiness Diet: A Nutritional Prescription for a Sharp Brain, Balanced Mood, and Lean, Energized Body* and *Fifty Shades of Kale: 50 Fresh and Satisfying Recipes That Are Bound to Please.*

We all know that a strong cup of coffee can give us that extra mental boost we may need to complete a brain-draining project or meet a tight deadline.

What works even better: Strategic eating is a healthful and reliable way to improve your ability to concentrate for the long haul—not just for a few hours at a time when you're hyped-up on caffeine.

There's no single food that will suddenly have you speed-reading a book in one sitting, but you can improve your overall powers of concentration by including the following foods in your diet…

• **Eggs.** When it comes to mental focus, it doesn't get much better than eggs! They're a leading source of a nutrient called choline, a precursor to the neurotransmitter acetylcholine—a key molecule of learning.

Eggs (including the yolks) also contain a variety of B vitamins, most of which have been stripped from the refined carbs that are so ubiquitous in the typical American diet. In particular, eggs are rich in vitamins B-6 and B-12, which are crucial for carrying out most cognitive functions (three large eggs will give you about half of your daily B-12 requirement)...and vitamin B-9 (also known as folate).

For optimal brain health, include up to 12 eggs in your diet each week. While cholesterol in one's diet has only a minimal effect on blood levels of cholesterol, consult your doctor for advice on appropriate intake of eggs if cholesterol is a concern.

•**Mussels.** Three ounces of mussels—which is a modest serving—contain 20 micrograms (mcg) of vitamin B-12 (that's nearly 10 times your daily requirement). Even a mild deficiency of this crucial brain-boosting vitamin can impair concentration and lead to fuzzy thinking.

But that's not all. Three ounces of mussels will also give you 430 mg of docosahexaenoic acid (DHA)—the equivalent of two to three typical fish oil supplement capsules. DHA is a type of omega-3 fatty acid needed for healthy brain function. Mussels are also loaded with zinc, a nutritional workhorse involved in more than 100 chemical reactions in the brain. Enjoy mussels twice a month.

Don't like mussels? Other smart brain-boosting seafood selections include oysters (six oysters deliver three to four times your daily zinc needs)...anchovies, which have more omega-3s than tuna...and clams, which are an excellent source of vitamin B-12.

Tasty choices: Caesar salad with anchovies...clam chowder...or pasta alle vongole (with clams).

• **Beef.** You've probably heard that eating too much red meat is linked to heart disease and even some types of cancer. However, you can minimize these risks and maximize your brainpower with a few small servings per week.

Here's why: Beef is a potent source of heme iron (the most absorbable form), which is needed to transport oxygen through the blood and to the brain.

What I recommend: Opt for grass-fed beef. It has fewer calories, less fat and more nutrients (such as vitamin E) than conventional beef. Meat from grass-fed animals has two to three times more conjugated linoleic acid (CLA) than meat from grain-fed animals. CLA helps protect the brain by counteracting the effects of harmful stress hormones.

Try to have grass-fed beef once or twice a week—but give it a supporting role instead of making it the star of your meal. Think grass-fed vegetable beef stew instead of a large steak.

Note: Even though grass-fed beef is more expensive than conventional beef, you can save by opting for nontraditional cuts, such as beef shank, stew meats and roasts. If you are a vegetarian or vegan, black beans are an excellent substitute.

•**Cruciferous vegetables.** Take your pick—the list includes brussels sprouts, kale, arugula, bok choy, cauliflower and collard greens. As members of the Brassica plant family, these veggies contain sulfur-based anti-inflammatory compounds that help protect the brain. One of these compounds, sulforaphane, has even been shown to improve memory and learning after brain injury.

Aim for at least two cups of cruciferous vegetables daily—I put that much in my kale-blueberry smoothie every morning!

Note: Consult your doctor before changing the amount of leafy greens you eat if you take warfarin, a blood thinner, since vitamin K–rich foods may interact.

Other good choices: Add purple cabbage to a stir-fry...or mash cauliflower instead of potatoes and season with brain-boosting turmeric and black pepper (to increase the absorption of turmeric).

Why Vegetarians Have It All Wrong

Terry Wahls, MD, an internist and a clinical professor of medicine at the University of Iowa Carver College of Medicine in Iowa City. She is author of *The Wahls Protocol: A Radical New Way to Treat All Chronic Autoimmune Conditions Using Paleo Principles* and founder of The Wahls Foundation, which educates the public and health-care practitioners on the benefits of integrative treatment for multiple sclerosis and other chronic diseases.

A diet rich in fruits and vegetables and whole grains, but with little or no meat, has long been touted as the best way to lower your risk for heart disease, prevent weight gain and reduce risk for certain cancers.

But as a medical doctor with progressive multiple sclerosis (MS), I believe that meat (grass-fed beef...organic chicken, pork and lamb...and wild game and fish) has played a critical role in my recovery—and that meat can help protect against other autoimmune diseases, Parkinson's disease, Alzheimer's disease and early cognitive impairment.

How Meat Benefits the Brain

•**Meat provides vitamin B-12.** A diet without meat raises your risk for vitamin B-12 deficiency. If your body doesn't get enough B-12, you can develop neurological symptoms such as problems with balance and coordination, difficulties with decision-making and cognitive decline. Vitamin B-12 is found naturally only in animal foods such as clams, liver, salmon and beef. A synthetic form is often added to cereals and nutritional yeast, but I recommend avoiding gluten because many people are sensitive to it. Alternatively, you could take a B-12 supplement, but I prefer natural food sources, which supply additional vitamins and nutrients.

•**Meat is the best source of complete proteins.** Protein is essential to make, repair and maintain the structure of all the cells in our bodies, including cells in the brain. The amino acids found in protein help the brain produce crucial neurotransmitters that regulate mood and maintain and repair brain cells. If you don't have enough protein to do this, brain function deteriorates.

Meat contains all of the essential amino acids your body needs to manufacture protein. To get a complete protein from a nonmeat source, you would have to combine a grain and a legume, for example.

•**Certain meats provide omega-3 fatty acids.** Cell membranes throughout the body, including in the brain, rely on essential fatty acids to stay healthy. The brain is especially dependent on the omega-3 fatty acids docosahexaenoic acid (DHA) and eicosapentaenoic acid (EPA) that are found in fish such as sardines, herring and anchovies (the fish I prefer to eat because small fish have less risk for heavy metal and plastic contamination) as well as organic chicken and grass-fed beef. These omega-3s help preserve the integrity of cell membranes in the brain and stave off neurological problems like mood disorders and cognitive decline.

While you can get alpha linolenic acid (ALA), another omega-3, from plant sources, your body can convert only small amounts of ALA into DHA and EPA. DHA and EPA supplements are available, but numerous studies have shown that foods high in omega-3s are more beneficial to brain health than supplements.

The Best Meat for Your Brain

Most grass-fed beef, organic chicken and wild game and fish are beneficial for brain health, but organ meats (particularly heart, liver and tongue) provide the most nutrition. Organ meats are chock-full of vitamins A and B and essential nutrients such as creatine, carnitine and coenzyme Q10 (CoQ10). There are a variety of ways to add organ meats to your meals and make them more palatable. *To get the most nutrition from meat…*

•**Start with heart.** Beef and bison heart taste a lot like steak, especially if you serve them up with mushrooms. Just don't overcook organ meat, or it will be dry and tough. Cooking it to medium rare also helps the meat retain vitamins.

•**Disguise liver.** If you don't like the taste of liver, purée small raw pieces of it in a blender with water to make a slurry. Add this mixture to soups, stews or chili, and let the food simmer a few minutes.

•**Try sausage or liver pâté.** Your local butcher can make a sausage out of ground liver and some other ground meat, such as pork or chicken. Start with a ratio of one part liver to six parts ground meat, and work up to a ratio of one to three. If you don't like the taste of liver, ask the butcher to add spices to conceal it.

•**Make a bone broth.** Put the carcass of a chicken or beef or pork knuckle bones into a pot. Add one tablespoon of vinegar per one quart of water, and toss in one whole onion and carrot and a few cloves of garlic. Let the broth simmer for at least six hours, then strain out the bone, vegetables and foam. Use the broth as a stock for soup or drink it.

•**Consider an organ meat supplement.** If you just can't stomach the idea of eating organ meat, consider taking a supplement.

Good choice: Organ Delight from Dr. Ron's Ultra-Pure (DrRons.com).

The Wahls Protocol

Keep in mind that I'm not advocating a meat-only diet. In fact, the Wahls Protocol diet (the eating plan I developed to combat my own MS) starts by recommending six to nine cups a day (depending on your size and gender) of vegetables, fruits and berries (get twice as many veggies as fruits and berries).

In particular, I prefer green, leafy vegetables…sulfur-rich vegetables in the cabbage and onion families…deeply colored vegetables such as yams, beets, peppers and tomatoes…and brightly colored berries such as raspberries, strawberries and cranberries.

For meat, I recommend six to 12 ounces a day (depending on your size and gender) for disease treatment and prevention.

My regimen also incorporates a CoQ10 supplement, a spirulina or chlorella algae supplement and green tea—which is high in quercetin, an antioxidant with anti-inflammatory properties.

Water Helps Your Brain

Daniel G. Amen, MD, a brain-imaging specialist and founder, CEO and medical director of the Amen Clinics. He is author of numerous books, including *Use Your Brain to Change Your Age*. AmenClinics.com

Drinking water is the easiest thing you can do for your brain, but most people don't drink anywhere near enough.

Fact: About 80% of the brain is comprised of water. If you don't drink enough—or if you drink a lot of dehydrating liquids, such as coffee or alcohol—you're going to struggle to think clearly and you may have memory problems. That's because dehydration increases stress hormones, and stress hormones interfere with cognitive abilities.

Recommended: Drink half your weight in water ounces every day.

Example: If you weigh 150 pounds, you'll want to drink 75 ounces of water a day. Drink more during the warm months or if you exercise regularly and lose water in perspiration.

Five Best Brain-Boosting Drinks

David Grotto, RD, a registered dietitian and founder and president of Nutrition House-call, LLC, a Chicago–based nutrition consulting firm. He is an adviser to *Fitness* magazine and blogs for the Real Life Nutrition community featured on WebMD. He is author of *The Best Things You Can Eat*.

Some of the easiest-to-prepare brain foods—meaning foods that can preserve and even improve your memory and other cognitive functions—are actually delicious drinks.

You probably already know about green tea, which is high in epigallocatechin-3-gallate (EGCG), a potent compound that appears to protect neurons from age-related damage. *But the following five drinks are scientifically proven to help your brain, too…*

Beet Juice

Beets are a nutritional powerhouse—and so is the juice. It increases levels of nitric oxide, a blood gas that improves blood flow. How does that help your brain? Your brain needs good blood flow to function optimally.

A recent study looked at brain scans of participants before and after they drank beet juice. The post-beverage scans showed an increase in circulation to the brain's white matter in the frontal lobes—a part of the brain that's often damaged in people with dementia.

You can buy ready-made beet juice at health-food stores, although it's much less expensive to make your own with fresh beets (include the root and greens, which are nutritious as well).

Beet juice has a naturally sweet taste, but you may want to add a little apple juice or another fruit juice—both for flavor and to make the mixture more pourable.

Berry Smoothies

Acai, a South American fruit that reduces inflammation, is ranked near the top of brain-healthy foods because it dilates blood vessels and increases blood flow.

Its juice has a pleasant taste—something like a cross between raspberry and cocoa—but it's very expensive (typically about $30 or more for a quart).

What I recommend: Blend a variety of everyday frozen berries that have been shown to boost brain health—raspberries, blueberries and strawberries, for example—along with a little acai juice (and a bit of any other fruit juice, if you wish) to make an easy, delicious smoothie.

Why use frozen berries? They retain the nutritional benefit of fresh berries—and they're easy to buy and last a long time in the freezer…they give your smoothie a nice texture, which you can vary by adding more or less juice…and they're less expensive than fresh berries if you buy large bags.

Carrot Juice

The old adage is that carrots are good for the eyes (indeed they are)—but we now know that carrot juice is absolutely great for the brain. Like other deeply colored vegetables (sweet potatoes, kale, red peppers, etc.), carrots are high in beta-carotene, an antioxidant that reduces inflammation—believed to be a factor in brain deterioration.

If you have tried carrot juice but didn't like the taste (it's surprisingly sweet), that's no problem. It is a very good "base" for multivegetable juices. (Some choices that are good for covering up the carrot flavor include kale, spinach and other dark greens.)

Cocoa

A Harvard/Brigham and Women's Hospital study found that adults who drank two daily cups of cocoa did better on memory tests than those who didn't drink it.

The flavanols (a class of antioxidants) in cocoa relax the endothelial linings of blood vessels and help reduce blood pressure. High blood pressure is a leading risk factor for dementia. The antioxidants in cocoa also reduce the cell-damaging effects of free radicals—this may improve long-term brain health.

Important: Do not go overboard with sugar, though—sugar is not good for your brain (and the jury is still out on artificial sweeteners).

Here's my advice: Buy a brand of unsweetened cocoa powder that is processed to remain high in flavanols. You don't have to buy an expensive specialty brand to get the brain-protecting effects. Most major brands of cocoa powder have respectable levels of cocoa flavanols. I advise against using milk chocolate or chocolate syrup—they typically have the least amount of flavanols and the most sugar.

At first, make your hot cocoa with your usual amount of sugar...then slowly cut back. You'll grow to appreciate the deep and pleasantly bitter true taste of the cocoa itself as less and less sugar stops masking it. As for using milk or water for your cocoa, that's your choice.

Seeds for Brain Health

Flaxseeds, sunflower seeds, sesame seeds and pumpkin seeds all contain high levels of polyunsaturated oils, as well as protein, vitamins and minerals—including magnesium, which is especially important for brain health.

Best: Nibble seeds instead of other snacks, or add them to salads. There is no need to measure them precisely—about three to four tablespoons a day is ideal.

Larry McCleary, MD, a retired pediatric neurosurgeon in Incline Village, Nevada, and author of *The Brain Trust Program.*

Red Wine

Everyone knows that red wine promotes cardiovascular health (easy does it). What you might not know is that red wine has been linked to a lower risk for dementia.

One reason is that people who drink moderate amounts of red wine—up to two glasses a day for men or one glass for women—have an increase in HDL "good" cholesterol. Research from Columbia University has found that people with the highest levels of HDL were less likely to develop dementia than those with the lowest levels.

Want to supercharge the brain-boosting power of your red wine? Make delicious Sangria! You'll get the wine's benefits and extra antioxidants and other nutrients from the fruit.

Sangria is typically made by steeping pieces of fresh fruit—lemon, orange, apple and just about any other fruit you like—in a rich red wine such as Merlot or Cabernet Sauvignon (or a Spanish red if you want to be auténtico) and adding sugar and another liquor, such as brandy or rum.

My advice: Skip the sugar and extra liquor, but go ahead and add some orange juice to dilute the wine a bit and add some sweetness.

Which Chocolate Is Best?

Bill Gottlieb, CHC, founder and president of Good For You Health Coaching, author of several books including *Health-Defense: How to Stay Vibrantly Healthy in a Toxic World* and *The Every-Other-Day Diet: The Diet That Lets You Eat All You Want (Half the Time) and Keep the Weight Off*, with Krista Varady, PhD. BillGottliebHealth.com

Nearly every client in my health-coaching practice gets a recommendation to consume a daily dose of about 400 milligrams (mg) of cocoa flavanols—the amount used in many of the studies that show a therapeutic effect.

Important: Higher doses don't produce better results.

And the healthiest way to get those flavanols is with unsweetened cocoa powder that delivers all the flavanols of dark chocolate without burdening your daily diet with extra calories and sugar. (Using cocoa powder also helps you control your intake—it's notoriously easy to consume an entire three-ounce bar of chocolate even though your optimal daily "dose" is only one ounce.)

Red flag: Do not use "Dutch" cocoa powder, which is treated with an alkalizing agent for a richer color and milder taste—a process that strips cocoa of 98% of its epicatechin.

My advice: Mix one tablespoon of unsweetened cocoa powder in an eight-to-12-ounce mug of hot water or milk (nondairy milks such as coco-

Olive Oil Helps Your Memory

Saturated fat, such as that found in meat and cheese, contributes to declines in memory and cognition—but monounsaturated fat, like that in olive oil, seems to protect the brain.

Recent study: Women over age 65 who ate the most saturated fat were up to 65% more likely to experience cognitive decline over time than those who ate the least. Women who ate the most monounsaturated fat were 44% less likely to decline in verbal-memory scores and 48% less likely to decline in overall cognition.

Olivia I. Okereke, MD, associate psychiatrist, Brigham and Women's Hospital, Boston, and leader of a study of 6,183 women, published in *Annals of Neurology.*

nut, almond, soy and rice milk are delicious alternatives) and add a no-calorie natural sweetener, such as stevia.

Good products: I recommend CocoaVia, the powder developed by Mars, Incoporated. The Mars Center for Cocoa Health Science has conducted extensive scientific research on cocoa flavanols for two decades, and one "stick" of its powder reliably delivers 375 mg of cocoa flavanols, standardized for epicatechin. You can mix it with cold or warm milk, coffee drinks, smoothies, yogurt or oatmeal. Another high-quality cocoa powder is CocoaWell from Reserveage. (*Note:* CocoaVia does process its products with alkali, but it's not a concern because the powder is reliably standardized to deliver a high, therapeutic dose of cocoa flavanols.)

Dark chocolate bars don't reliably deliver a therapeutic dose of cocoa flavanols. But if you prefer to eat dark chocolate, look for a bar with 70% or more cocoa, and consume about one ounce (28 grams) per day. According to a report from ConsumerLab.com, dark chocolate brands with high levels of flavanols (about one-quarter to one-half the amount in the best brands of cocoa powder) include Endangered Species, Ghirardelli and Lindt.

Green Tea Boosts Brain Power

Qi Dai, MD, PhD, professor of medicine, division of general internal medicine and public health, Vanderbilt School of Medicine, Nashville, and leader of a study of 1,836 people of Japanese descent, published in *The American Journal of Medicine.*

In a recent Japanese study of cognitive function in people age 70 or older, participants who drank two or more cups of green tea daily had a 54% lower prevalence of cognitive decline—measured via memory, attention and language-use tests—than those who drank three cups or less weekly.

Theory: Antioxidants in green tea may reduce the buildup of a type of plaque in the brain that is responsible for memory loss in Alzheimer's disease.

Self-defense: Drink two or more cups of green tea daily to help promote brain health.

Sage for the Brain

Bill Gottlieb, CHC, editor of *Healing Spices: How to Use 50 Everyday and Exotic Spices to Boost Health and Beat Disease,* founder and president of Good For You Health Coaching, former editor in chief of Rodale Books and Prevention Magazine Health Books and author of numerous health books that have sold more than two million copies. BillGottliebHealth.com

The botanical name for sage—Salvia officinalis—comes from the Latin salvare, meaning "to save" or "to cure." *And sage lives up to its name…*

•**Memory problems.** One hour after people took a supplement of sage oil, they had better memory, more focused attention and more alertness, reported researchers in *Journal of Psychopharmacology.* In another study, people who smelled sage had a stronger memory and were in a better mood.

•**Anxiety.** In a study published in *Neuropsychopharmacology,* people who took a supplement of dried sage leaf were less anxious and felt calmer and more content than when they took a placebo.

Why it works: Sage may block the action of cholinesterase, an enzyme that destroys acetylcholine, a brain chemical that plays a role in memory, attention and alertness. Sage also might improve the functioning of cholinergic receptors on brain cells that receive acetylcholine.

How to use sage: Because of its robust flavor, sage is best used in hearty dishes such as pot roast, meat loaf and stuffing. It also goes well with squash, sweet potatoes and apples.

However: The amounts that improve mental and emotional functioning aren't easy to get with diet, so you may want to take a sage leaf supplement. I often recommend the herbal extract from Herb Pharm because it's made from the whole leaf that has been grown organically. Follow the directions on the label.

For a Quick Memory Booster, Grab a Cup of Joe

Study participants given 200 milligrams (mg) of caffeine in tablet form—the amount of caffeine contained in a strong cup of coffee—performed better on a memory test than people who were not given caffeine. In the test, participants had to identify pictures that were slightly different from ones they had seen the day before.

Study of 160 people, ages 18 to 30, none of whom consumed caffeine on a regular basis, by researchers at Johns Hopkins University, Baltimore, published in *Nature Neuroscience.*

Turmeric: The Spice That May Prevent Alzheimer's

Mark A. Stengler, NMD, a naturopathic doctor and founder of the Stengler Center for Integrative Medicine in Encinitas, California. He is author or coauthor of numerous books, including *The Natural Physician's Healing Therapies* and *Bottom Line's Prescription for Natural Cures*, and author of the newsletter *Health Revelations*. MarkStengler.com

In India, the smell of turmeric, the bright yellow spice used in curries, fills almost every restaurant and home. Indians eat turmeric because they like it, but rapidly growing evidence indicates that the spice is giving them much more than flavor.

Thousands of years ago, Ayurvedic and traditional Chinese medicine recognized turmeric as a healing agent for everything from flatulence to liver disease. Now modern research demonstrates that properties in this zesty spice may be useful for lowering rates of breast, prostate, lung and colon cancers, and also for treating breast cancer, inflammatory bowel disease, Crohn's disease and possibly cystic fibrosis.

But even newer and especially exciting research concerns the relationship between turmeric and Alzheimer's disease. Nearly 10 years ago, researchers in India became curious about the influence turmeric might have on rates of Alzheimer's. They looked to see how many people over age 65 in a town in India had signs of the disease, versus a similar group of people in a similar-sized Pennsylvania town, where most people eat little—or no—turmeric.

What they found: In India, just 4.7 per 1,000 person-years (a common measure of incidence rate) showed signs of Alzheimer's, compared with a rate of 17.5 per 1,000 person-years in Pennsylvania. In fact, India has among the lowest rates of Alzheimer's disease in the world. Another study, from the National University of Singapore, involved 1,010 people over age 60. Those who reported that they ate curry "often or very often" or even "occasionally" scored higher on mental performance tests than those who rarely or never consumed it.

What Is Turmeric?

Turmeric is a powder made from the root of the plant Curcuma longa, which grows in southern Asia. The part of the plant that is responsible for healing is the yellow pigment, called curcumin.

When it comes to health-giving properties, curcumin gives twice. It is a potent anti-inflammatory agent, without the potential side effects of anti-inflammatory drugs. These include damage to the lining of the stomach and intestines and a greater risk for kidney and liver problems, heart attack and stroke. Next, curcumin is a powerful antioxidant—it tracks down and reduces free radicals, insidious molecules that otherwise would cause damage in the body. Both of these properties are important when it comes to preventing or slowing the progression of Alzheimer's disease.

In healthy people, immune cells attack and destroy amyloid-beta plaques—a buildup of proteins between neurons in the brain. But in people with Alzheimer's, this immune response is less efficient and allows plaques to form. Plaque triggers inflammation and free radicals, both of which cause cell damage in the brain. Curcumin slows this harmful process in a number of ways—it forms a powerful bond with the amyloid protein that prevents the protein from clumping...it may break down plaques as well, preliminary research demonstrates...and finally, as I noted before, curcumin reduces the oxidative damage and brain inflammation that are linked to Alzheimer's disease.

Cholesterol Blaster

There is yet more good news about curcumin's power to prevent and even fight Alzheimer's disease. Elevated cholesterol is thought to be involved in the development of Alzheimer's—and studies demonstrate that curcumin reduces cholesterol. In one study, healthy volunteers took 500 mg of curcumin supplements every day for one week.

Result: Reduced levels of total cholesterol and also lipid peroxides (markers of free radical damage to fats).

Spice Up Your Diet

In the meantime, I encourage all my patients, especially those over age 50, to consume one or two teaspoons a day of turmeric. There are many ways to incorporate this spice into your regular diet. You can sprinkle it into egg salad or over vegetables while sautéing...add it to soups or broths...put it on fish or meat...and use it to flavor rice or a creamy vegetable dip. And of course, turmeric adds zing to curries. If you want to make the most healthful curry dishes, it is important to purchase turmeric as a separate spice—lab tests show that many curry powders in this country contain almost no turmeric.

Anyone taking blood-thinning drugs should discuss using turmeric or curcumin supplements with a doctor, because curcumin is a natural blood thinner. Turmeric also can cause gallbladder contractions, so those with a history of gallstones or gallbladder problems also should consult a doctor. There is no risk in mixing curcumin with pharmaceutical drugs for Alzheimer's disease.

Rosemary for Better Memory

Ann Kulze, MD, a primary care physician and founder and CEO of Just Wellness, LLC. She is author of *Dr. Ann's 10-Step Diet: A Simple Plan for Permanent Weight Loss and Lifelong Vitality.* DrAnnsWellness.com

It turns out that Shakespeare's Ophelia wasn't all that far off when she said that rosemary is for remembrance. According to a study in *Journal of Neurochemistry*, rosemary contains the compound carnosic acid (CA), which helps protect the brain.

This savory herb also contains phytochemicals that can reduce the formation of cancer-causing compounds known as heterocyclic amines (HCAs). HCAs can form when the proteins in meat are heated to high temperatures.

Preliminary research also indicates that rosemary may enhance insulin sensitivity, improving the action and efficiency of insulin in the body, aiding in a healthy metabolism and slowing the aging process.

Suggested uses: I always add one teaspoon of dried rosemary or a tablespoon or two of fresh to a pound of ground meat before grilling burgers. Rosemary also is good in lamb and potato dishes, soups and stews.

The Most Powerful Brain-Building Nutrients and Herbs

Mao Shing Ni ("Dr. Mao"), PhD, DOM (doctor of oriental medicine), **LAc** (licensed acupuncturist), chancellor and cofounder of Yo San University in Los Angeles, and codirector of Tao of Wellness, a clinic in Santa Monica, California. He is author of numerous books, including *Second Spring: Dr. Mao's Hundreds of Natural Secrets for Women to Revitalize and Regenerate at Any Age.* TaoOfWellness.com

Cognitive declines can result from hormonal changes and reductions in neurotransmitters, chemicals that help brain cells communicate with each other. Increasing your intake of certain nutrients helps balance hormones and protect neurotransmitters.

Ask your doctor before supplementing, especially if you have a health condition...use medication...or are pregnant or breast-feeding. To reduce the risk for interactions, do not take supplements within 30 minutes of medication... and limit your use of these supplements to any four of the following.

Nutrients Your Mind Needs

For the foods recommended below, one serving equals four ounces of meat, poultry, fish, or soy products...eight ounces of milk...two ounces of nuts... two eggs (with yolks)...one-half cup of vegetables or fruit...and one cup of leafy greens.

•**Choline.** The neurotransmitter acetylcholine plays a key role in learning and memory. Choline is a precursor to acetylcholine that is produced in the liver. Production of choline declines with age, as does the body's ability to efficiently use the choline that remains.

Brain boost: Eat one or more servings daily of choline-rich broccoli, cauliflower, eggs, kidney beans, navy beans, liver, milk or peanuts.

Supplement option: 1,200 milligrams (mg) daily.

•**DMAE (2-dimethylaminoethanol).** The body uses fatty acids to create brain cells and neurotransmitters. DMAE, a chemical in fatty acids, helps produce acetylcholine.

Brain boost: Have two servings weekly of DMAE-rich anchovies or sardines. If fresh fish is not available, have canned water-packed sardines or anchovies and rinse before eating to reduce salt.

Supplement option: 500 mg twice daily after meals.

•**L-carnitine.** Mitochondria are the engines of cells. The amino acid L-carnitine transports fatty acids to mitochondria for use as fuel and provides nutrients to brain cells.

Brain boost: Have two weekly servings of lamb or poultry, which are rich in L-carnitine.

Supplement option: 500 mg to 1,000 mg before breakfast and again in the afternoon.

•**Vitamin B-12.** This is key to red blood cell formation and nerve cell health. The body's ability to absorb vitamin B-12 diminishes with age—about 10% to 15% of people over age 60 are deficient in it.

Brain boost: Have two servings weekly of beef or lamb...halibut, salmon, sardines or sea bass...eggs...or vitamin B-12–enriched soybean products (miso, tempeh).

Supplement option: 500 micrograms (mcg) to 1,000 mcg daily.

The Most Helpful Herbs

An easy way to get the benefits of mind-sharpening herbs is to brew them into a tisane, or herbal infusion—more commonly called herbal tea.

To brew: Pour eight ounces of very hot water over one heaping tablespoon of fresh herbs or one teaspoon of dried herbs. Steep for five minutes, strain and drink.

Convenient: To reduce the number of cups needed to meet the daily recommendations below, brew two or more herbs together.

●**Chinese club moss.** This herb contains the chemical huperzine A, which helps conserve acetylcholine.

Brain boost: Drink one to two cups of Chinese club moss tea each day.

Supplement option: 50 mcg of huperzine A twice daily (discontinue if supplements cause gastric upset or hyperactivity).

●**Ginkgo biloba.** This herb increases blood flow to the brain's tiny capillaries and combats DNA damage caused by free radicals.

Caution: Do not use ginkgo if you take blood-thinning medication, such as *warfarin* (Coumadin).

Brain boost: Drink three cups of ginkgo tea daily.

Supplement option: 120 mg daily.

●**Kitchen herbs. Oregano,** peppermint, rosemary and sage have oils that may increase blood flow in the brain and/or support neurotransmitters, promoting alertness.

Brain boost: Use any or all of these herbs to brew a cup of tea for a pick-me-up in the morning and again in the afternoon.

Also: Use herbs liberally when cooking.

Supplement option: About 150 mg each of any or all of these herbs daily, alone or in combination.

●**Mugwort (wormwood).** This herb improves circulation, aiding delivery of nutrients to brain cells.

Brain boost: Twice a week, drink one cup of mugwort tea…add a half-dozen leaves of fresh mugwort to salad…or sauté leaves with garlic or onions.

Supplement option: 300 mg daily.

Caution: Avoid mugwort during pregnancy—it may stimulate uterine contractions.

D: The Memory Vitamin

Daniel G. Amen, MD, a brain-imaging specialist and medical director of Amen Clinics, Inc., based in Newport Beach, California. He is author of numerous books, including *Use Your Brain to Change Your Age.* AmenClinics.com

Americans don't get enough sun, and because of this, about two-thirds of adults don't meet their vitamin D needs through sunshine exposure. You probably know that vitamin D is essential for bone strength as well as for preventing some cancers, including breast cancer.

What's new: Vitamin D appears to help the immune system remove beta-amyloid, an abnormal protein, from the brain. This is important because beta-amyloid causes the "tangles" that are associated with Alzheimer's disease.

Brain cells use vitamin D for learning, memory and other cognitive functions. It also is an antioxidant that protects neurons from cell-damaging inflammation. A Tufts University study found that elderly adults with optimal levels of vitamin D performed better on cognitive tests and had better brain-processing speeds than those with lower levels.

Recommended: 2,000 international units (IU) of vitamin D daily is a typical dose, but I advise patients to get their blood levels of vitamin D tested before taking supplements. Everyone synthesizes and absorbs vitamin D differently.

Stop Memory Loss with Doctor-Tested Supplements

Pamela W. Smith, MD, MPH, codirector of the master's program in metabolic and nutritional medicine at Morsani College of Medicine at University of South Florida and owner/director of the Michigan-based Center for Personalized Medicine. She is author of *What You Must Know About Memory Loss & How You Can Stop It: A Guide to Proven Techniques and Supplements to Maintain, Strengthen, or Regain Memory.* CFHLL.com

Mild forgetfulness, known as age-related memory impairment, is a natural part of getting older. By age 75, a person's memory has declined, on average, by about 43%. After age 75, the hippocampus, the part of the brain most closely associated with memory, will eventually atrophy at the rate of 1% to 2% each year.

But you can improve memory with over-the-counter supplements—if you choose the right ones. Here are the supplements I find most effective with my patients. You can take several of these if you choose. You could start with phosphatidylserine and add others depending on your personal needs. For example, if you're taking a medication that depletes CoQ10, you might want to take that supplement. Or if you're under stress, add ashwagandha root. Of course, always check with your doctor before starting any new supplement.

•**Phosphatidylserine (PS).** Most people haven't heard of it, but PS is one of my first choices for mild memory loss. It's a naturally occurring phospholipid (a molecule that contains two fatty acids) that increases the body's production of acetylcholine and other neurotransmitters. It improves cell-to-cell communication and "nourishes" the brain by improving glucose metabolism.

Studies have shown that healthy people who take PS are more likely to maintain their ability to remember things. For those who have already experienced age-related memory loss, PS can improve memory. It's also thought to improve symptoms caused by some forms of dementia.

Typical dose: 300 mg daily. You're unlikely to notice any side effects.

•**Co-enzyme Q10 (CoQ10).** This is another naturally occurring substance found in many foods (such as fatty fish, meats, nuts, fruits and vegetables) and in nearly all of your body's tissues. CoQ10 increases the production of adenosine triphosphate, a molecule that enhances energy production within cells. It's also a potent antioxidant that reduces cell-damaging inflammation in the brain and other parts of the body.

People with degenerative brain disorders, such as Alzheimer's, tend to have lower levels of CoQ10. Studies suggest that supplemental CoQ10 improves memory by protecting brain cells from oxidative damage.

Important: If you're taking a medication that depletes CoQ10—examples include statins (for lowering cholesterol)…metformin (for diabetes)…and beta-blockers (for heart disease and other conditions)—you'll definitely want to take a supplement. I often recommend it for people age 50 and older because the body's production of CoQ10 declines with age. Hard exercise also depletes it.

Typical dose: Between 30 mg and 360 mg daily. Ask your health-care professional how much you need—it will depend on medication use and other factors. Side effects are rare but may include insomnia, agitation and digestive problems such as diarrhea and heartburn.

•**Acetyl-L-carnitine.** A study that looked at people with mild cognitive impairment (an intermediate stage between age-related memory impairment and dementia) found that acetyl-L-carnitine improved memory, attention and even verbal fluency.

Acetyl-L-carnitine (it is derived from an amino acid) is a versatile molecule. It's used by the body to produce acetylcholine, the main neurotransmitter involved in memory. It slows the rate of neurotransmitter decay, increases oxygen availability and helps convert body fat into energy.

Typical dose: 1,000 mg to 2,000 mg daily. Check with your health-care professional before starting acetyl-L-carnitine to see what dose is best for you. If your kidneys are not functioning perfectly, you may need a lower dose. Some people may notice a slight fishy body odor. In my experience, you can prevent this by taking 50 mg to 100 mg of vitamin B-2 at the same time you take acetyl-L-carnitine.

•**Ashwagandha root.** This is an herb that improves the repair and regeneration of brain cells (neurons) and inhibits the body's production of acetylcholinesterase, an enzyme that degrades acetylcholine. It also improves the ability to deal with both physical and emotional stress—both of which have been linked to impaired memory and cognitive decline.

Typical dose: 500 mg to 2,000 mg daily. Start with the lower dose. If after a month you don't notice that your memory and focus have improved, take a little more. GI disturbances are possible but not common.

Warning: Don't take this supplement if you're also taking a prescription medication that has cholinesterase-inhibiting effects, such as donepezil (Aricept) or galantamine (Razadyne). Ask your health-care professional whether any of your medications have this effect.

•**Ginkgo biloba.** Among the most studied herbal supplements, ginkgo is an antioxidant that protects the hippocampus from age-related atrophy. It's a vasodilator that helps prevent blood clots, improves brain circulation and reduces the risk for vascular dementia, a type of dementia associated with impaired blood flow to the brain. It also increases the effects of serotonin, a neurotransmitter that's involved in mood and learning.

Bonus: In animal studies, ginkgo appears to block the formation of amyloid, the protein that has been linked to Alzheimer's disease. There's strong evidence that ginkgo can stabilize and possibly improve memory.

Typical dose: 60 mg to 120 mg daily. Most people won't have side effects, but ginkgo is a blood thinner that can react with other anticoagulants. If you're taking warfarin or another blood thinner (including aspirin and fish oil), be sure to check with your health-care professional before taking ginkgo.

•**Fish oil.** Much of the brain consists of DHA (docosahexaenoic acid), one of the main omega-3 fatty acids. It is essential for brain health. People who take fish-oil supplements have improved brain circulation and a faster transmission of nerve signals.

Studies have found that people who eat a lot of fatty fish have a lower risk for mild cognitive impairment than people who tend to eat little or no fatty fish. One study found that people with age-related memory impairment achieved better scores on memory tests when they took daily DHA supplements.

Typical dose: 2,000 mg daily if you're age 50 or older. Look for a combination supplement that includes equal amounts of DHA and EPA (another omega-3). Fish-oil supplements can increase the effects of blood-thinning medications such as aspirin and warfarin if the dose is above 3,000 mg a day.

•**Huperzine A.** Extracted from a Chinese moss, this is a cholinesterase inhibitor that increases brain levels of acetylcholine. It also protects brain cells from too-high levels of glutamate, another neurotransmitter.

Huperzine A may improve memory and could even help delay symptoms of Alzheimer's disease. A study conducted by the National Institute on Aging found that patients with mild-to-moderate Alzheimer's who took huperzine A had improvements in cognitive functions.

Recommended dose: 400 mcg daily. Don't take it if you're already taking a prescription cholinesterase inhibitor (as discussed in the "Ashwagandha root" section).

The Ten Very Best Foods to Prevent Depression (and Build a Healthier Brain)

Drew Ramsey, MD, psychiatrist, Columbia University Medical Center, and assistant professor, Columbia University College of Physicians and Surgeons, both in New York City. His latest book is *Eat Complete*. DrewRamseyMD.com

Here's a startling statistic—studies show that people who consume a healthy diet are 40% to 50% less likely to develop depression.

What are the absolutely best nutrients—and most nutrient-packed foods—to protect your brain from depression and other ailments?

What protects mood also protects against dementia and other brain-related conditions. The brain is the biggest asset we have, so we should be selecting foods that specifically nourish the brain.

Here's how to build the healthiest brain possible—starting in your kitchen.

Nutrients Brains Need Most

These key nutrients as the most important…

•**Long-chain omega-3 fatty acids.** There are two major ones. Docosahexaenoic acid (DHA) creates hormones called "neuroprotectins and resolvins" that combat brain inflammation, which is implicated in the development of depression (as well as dementia). Eicosapentaenoic acid (EPA) protects the cardiovascular system, important for a healthy brain.

•**Zinc.** This mineral plays a major role in the development of new brain cells and can boost the efficacy of antidepressant medications.

•**Folate.** Also known as vitamin B-9, folate is needed for good moods and a healthy brain. It helps produce defensin-1, a molecule that protects the brain and increases the concentration of acetylcholine, a neurotransmitter that's crucial to memory and cognition.

•**Iron.** This essential element is a crucial cofactor in the synthesis of mood-regulating neurotransmitters including dopamine and serotonin.

•**Magnesium.** This mineral is required to keep myelin—the insulation of brain cells—healthy. It also increases brain-derived neurotrophic factor (BDNF), which promotes the growth of new neurons and healthy connections among brain cells. A deficiency in magnesium can lead to depression, anxiety, symptoms of ADHD, insomnia and fatigue.

Try Bacopa for Memory Loss

This herbal medicine contains bacosides, compounds that appear to improve the repair, production and signaling of nerve cells. A 12-week study found that people who took 300 mg of Bacopa daily had improvements in memory and information processing.

Typical dose: To help protect your memory, take 300 mg daily. Look for a product that contains 50% bacosides. Take it with food to help avoid stomach upset.

Mark A. Moyad, MD, MPH, director of preventive and alternative medicine at the University of Michigan Medical Center. He is also the author, with Janet Lee, of *The Supplement Handbook.*

•**Vitamin B-12.** This vitamin, which often is deficient as we age, helps makes neurotransmitters that are key to mood and memory.

•**Vitamin E.** This potent antioxidant vitamin protects polyunsaturated fatty acids in the brain—including DHA. Vitamin E–rich foods, but not supplements, are linked to the prevention of clinical depression as well as slower progression of Alzheimer's disease. One reason may be that most supplements contain only alpha-tocopherol, while other vitamin E compounds, particularly tocotrienols, play important roles in brain function.

•**Dietary fiber.** A high-fiber diet supports healthy gut bacteria (the gut "microbiome"), which growing evidence suggests is key for mental health.

Boosting Your Mood at the Supermarket

The best brain foods are mostly plant-based, but seafood, wild game and even some organ meats make the top of the list, too...

•**Leafy greens such as kale, mustard greens and collard greens**

•**Bell peppers such as red, green and orange**

•**Cruciferous vegetables such as cauliflower, broccoli and cabbage**

•**Berries such as strawberries, raspberries and blueberries**

•**Nuts such as pecans, walnuts, almonds and cashews**

•**Bivalves such as oysters, clams and mussels**

•**Crustaceans such as crab, lobster and shrimp**

•**Fish such as sardines, salmon and fish roe**

•**Organ meats such as liver, poultry giblets and heart**

•**Game and wild meat such as bison, elk and duck**

Eating these nutrient-dense foods is likely to help prevent and treat mental illness. When someone with depression is treated, the real goal is to prevent that person from ever getting depressed again.

Everyday Brain Foods

Not into eating beef heart? Having a little trouble stocking up on elk? When it comes to meat, wild game may not be widely available, but grass-fed beef, which is higher in omega-3 fatty acids than conventionally raised beef, is stocked in most supermarkets—and may be independently associated with protection from depression.

Other foods that didn't make it to the top of the Brain Food Scale but that still are very good for the brain include eggs (iron, zinc), beans (fiber, magnesium, iron) and fruits and vegetables of all colors (fiber, antioxidants). Plus, small quantities of dark chocolate, which gives you a little dopamine rush. Dopamine, he explains, is a neurotransmitter that provides a feeling of reward.

Lecithin for Poor Memory

C. Norman Shealy, MD, PhD, founder and CEO of the International Institute of Holistic Medicine. He is author of many books, including *The Healing Remedies Sourcebook*. NormShealy.com

Lecithin is the common name for a group of related chemical compounds known as phosphatidylcholine. It's converted in the body into acetylcholine, a neurotransmitter that plays a critical role in many brain functions, including memory. One study found that participants who took two tablespoons of lecithin daily for five weeks had fewer memory lapses and performed better on memory tests than those who took a placebo.

How to use it: Take two heaping tablespoons of the granules twice daily. I put it in water, but it can be mixed in food, juice or milk. There are no side effects associated with this dose.

Chromium and Memory

Robert Krikorian, PhD, professor of clinical psychiatry, University of Cincinnati, Ohio.

When 26 adults with mild memory loss took a 1,000-mcg chromium picolinate supplement or a placebo daily for 12 weeks, the supplement group performed better on memory tests while the placebo group showed no change.

Theory: This trace mineral reduces insulin resistance, a condition in which the body's cells don't use insulin properly. Too little insulin in the brain may contribute to poor memory.

If you're concerned about your memory: Ask your doctor about taking 400 mcg of chromium picolinate daily.

Caution: This supplement may affect dosage requirements for diabetes medications.

CHAPTER 8

Memory Boosters

Best Techniques to Improve Your Memory

Gary Small, MD, director of the Longevity Center at the Semel Institute for Neuroscience & Human Behavior, University of California, Los Angeles. He is also coauthor of many books, including *iBrain, Snap! Change Your Personality in 30 Days* and *2 Weeks to a Younger Brain*. DrGarySmall.com

Age is the biggest factor for memory loss. We all have memory problems of some sort by age 60, such as momentarily forgetting someone's name, or briefly wondering why we just walked into a room. We can't stop the effects of aging, but we can slow them down.

Using very simple techniques and lifestyle changes—such as reading regularly and playing board games—can have a positive impact on memory retention. Scientific research shows that whenever we push ourselves to solve problems in a new way, we may be strengthening the connections between our brain cells.

Memory Techniques

Some people are so good at memorizing things that they test their talent in competitive matches involving knowledge of trivia or the recall of remarkably large numbers. Scientists have found that those people are no different from the rest of us. There is nothing out of the ordinary in their brain structure nor are there any indications of unusual intelligence. They simply often tap into a memory technique used since antiquity called the Roman Room method.

This method is simple. Visualize yourself walking a familiar route, such as the rooms of your home. Mentally place images of the items to be remembered on specific points on the route. It may be helpful to place items where they may logically be—if you want to remember to buy coffee beans, perhaps they're best mentally placed on the kitchen counter. When you want to recall them, mentally retrace your steps.

Over time, you can add more objects to the rooms. If one day you want to remember to pick up the newspaper, add it next to the coffee beans on the counter. If it's airline tickets, visualize them taped to the fridge door. You can also extend your route or even add other familiar locations for certain kinds of memory tasks.

The Roman Room method is a very useful technique. Orators back in Ancient Rome would remember lengthy speeches this way, imagining each progression of a speech by mentally walking through rooms where they had placed objects to remind themselves of lines. *Yet since today we have much more clutter coming at us, I also teach my patients an additional memory technique that I call look, snap, connect...*

•**Look reminds us to focus our attention.** The most common explanation for memory loss is that the information never gets into our minds in the first place. Because we are distracted, we don't take in the information or don't allow ourselves to absorb it. Simply reminding ourselves to focus our attention will dramatically boost memory power.

•**Snap stands for creating a mental snapshot or visual image in your mind's eye of the information to be remembered.** For most people, visual images are much easier to remember than other forms of information.

•**Connect means we need to link up the visual images from snap in meaningful ways.** These associations are key to recalling memories when we want them later. When linking your mental images, create a story that has action and detail.

Example: Say that you want to remember five words on your "to do" list: mail, gasoline, grandson, sweater, airline. Come up with a story linking them. For instance, I imagine a grandson knitting a sweater on a plane, then mailing it at the airport, when the plane lands to refuel.

Whatever the story ends up being, having detail, action and, for me, humor, all help to imprint the information.

This linking technique works very well with everyday memory tasks, such as grocery lists or errands to run.

When trying to remember faces and names, create an image either linked to the person whose name you need to remember or a distinguishing feature of his/her face. A redhead named Lucy could be remembered by noting that the red hair reminds you of Lucille Ball. You could remember the last name of a woman named Potvin by imagining that she landscaped her yard with pots full of vines.

Mental Aerobics

It's never too late to improve your memory. Recent studies show that even people in the early stages of Alzheimer's can be taught significant face and name retention under the guidance of a professional. For those of us looking to overcome the common forgetfulness in daily life, we can tackle much of that ourselves by doing activities that involve lateral thinking.

Lateral thinking means that we are trying to solve a problem from many angles instead of tackling it head on. *Here are some mental aerobic exercises to get you started and, hopefully, suggest further how to invoke lateral thinking in your life...*

Quiz Time

A lot of memory loss is simply being too busy to absorb what people are saying. These exercises are meant to remind you to slow down, pay attention and consider what is at hand. In doing so, your memory will improve...

1. Brush your hair using your nondominant hand. You may find it awkward at first, but over a few days notice how much easier it gets. This and other exercises don't directly help your memory (after all, how often will any of us need to remember to brush with the opposite hand?). What these mental aerobics do is challenge your mind to think differently and examine tasks we often do without thinking, and which lead to our minds getting "flabby."

2. Fill in a grid so that every row, column and two-by-two box contains the numbers 1, 2, 3 and 4.

3. Say "silk" six times. Then answer the following question: What do cows drink?

This exercise will help you be more thoughtful about things, which in turn is conducive to better memory.

4. See how many words you can spell from these letters: LIGOBATE.

No letter may be used twice in any given word, and each word must contain the letter L.

5. How many months have 28 days?

6. All of the vowels have been removed from the following saying. The remaining consonants are in the correct sequence, broken into groups of two to five letters. What is the saying?

STRK WHLTH RNS HT…

How well did you do? Regardless, this is just a start to remembering more and living better.

ANSWERS TO QUIZ…

Q2: Across row 1: 1, 2, 3, 4 or 1, 2, 4, 3. Row 2: 4, 3, 1, 2. Row 3: 2, 1, 4, 3 or 2, 1, 3, 4. Row 4: 3, 4, 2, 1.

Q3: Cows drink water. If you said "milk," you need to focus your attention.

Q4: able, agile, ail, alto, bagel, bail, bale, belt, bile, bilge, bleat, blog, boil, bolt, el, gable, Gail, gale, gel, gelato, gilt, glib, gloat, glob, globe, goal, goalie, lab, lag, late, lea, leg, let, lib, lie, lit, lob, lobe, log, loge, lot, oblate, obligate, oblige, ogle, oil, table, tail, tale, teal, tile, toil, toile.

Q5: All of them. (If you say only one month has 28 days, it's an example of not paying attention to the matter at hand—all months have 28 days, after all.)

Q6: Strike while the iron is hot.

Boost Your Memory in Minutes— (and Have Fun Doing It)

Cynthia R. Green, PhD, founder and president of Memory Arts, LLC, a memory fitness and brain-health consulting service in Montclair, New Jersey, and founding director of the Memory Enhancement Program at Mount Sinai School of Medicine in New York City. She is author of *Total Memory Workout: 8 Easy Steps to Maximum Memory Fitness.* TotalBrainHealth.com

We all have heard that the brain, like a muscle, requires regular mental exercise to stay fit. Most people assume that this means hard exercise—learning a new language, attending university classes, etc.

There are easier ways. I recommend fun and simple mental stretch activities that force the brain to look at the world in new ways. These "brain workouts" immediately exercise the brain and help you stay mentally sharp and agile, improving both memory and thinking skills.

Bonus: Similar types of brain workouts can help prevent later-life cognitive declines. A New England Journal of Medicine study found that people who spent the most time engaged in mentally stimulating activities, such as playing board games and writing for pleasure, were 63% less likely to develop dementia than those who did the least. *Activities to try…*

• **Tap a tune.** While imagining your favorite song, drum your fingers on a table or desktop to re-create the notes you are hearing in your head. This encourages the brain to coordinate memory, movement and auditory skills.

Expressing yourself this way cross-challenges the brain and causes it to activate different neural networks than the ones it normally uses.

• **Rework a word.** Write down a multisyllable word, such as "resolution," "sufficient" or "beneficence." Then see how many other words you can come up with, using the letters of the original word. This exercise forces you to see familiar things (the original word) in new ways. You can make it harder by giving yourself only two minutes to do the "word search." Timed activities encourage the use of different mental skills, such as speed, attention and flexibility.

• **Juggle.** Some of the best mental activities also have a physical component. German researchers found that complex motor integration activities, such as juggling, increased the brain's white matter, tissue that is composed of nerve fibers that transmit information to different areas of the brain.

You can learn basic juggling techniques by watching Internet videos.

Helpful: Start with juggling lightweight scarves. They're easier for beginners to juggle than, say, tennis balls.

• **Wear your watch upside down.** Can you tell what time it is when the numbers on your watch are reversed? It's harder than you think. This type of subtle change forces your brain to practice neurobics, activities that engage your attention and involve using one or more of your senses in a new way.

Another example: Using your non-dominant hand to brush your teeth. It takes practice!

• **Doodle.** Doodling does more than keep your hands busy. Using a pen or colored pencils to doodle or draw can change the ways in

Handwriting Is Healthy

Handwriting boosts learning and memory. Physically drawing letters activates a distinct neural pathway that improves reading comprehension and memory of language.

Claudia Aguirre, PhD, neuroscientist and mind-body expert based in the Los Angeles area, writing at HuffingtonPost.com.

Quick Memory Trick

For an easy trick to help you remember, close your eyes.

Recent research: Adults who closed their eyes after watching videos of crime reenactments had 23% better recall of what they'd seen and heard than those who kept their eyes open.

Explanation: Closing your eyes helps block distractions, improves focus and helps you visualize what you're trying to remember about past events and experiences.

Robert A. Nash, PhD, senior lecturer in psychology, Aston University, Birmingham, UK.

which you see your environment. It also requires mental focus to look closely at what's around you.

Better Brain Health Found in Bookworms

Robert Wilson, PhD, senior neuropsychologist, Rush Alzheimer's Disease Center, Chicago.

Memory and thinking tests given to approximately 300 adults revealed that those who participated in reading, writing and similar activities throughout their lives had a 32% lower rate of memory decline than those who did not. Reading helps strengthen circuits in the cerebral cortex, making them more resilient. The brain needs exercise just like other body parts, so keep it in shape at any age with mentally challenging activities, such as reading and/or writing.

Leave Your Memory at the Door

Gabriel Radvansky, PhD, professor, department of psychology, University of Notre Dame, Notre Dame, Indiana. He has been researching how memory works for most of his career.

How many times has something like this happened to you? While brushing your teeth, you remember an important phone call that you need to make as soon as you're done. But by the time you have finished brushing, you walk out of the bathroom, grab your coat and car keys and head out the door... totally forgetting all about that call that you really needed to make.

We all do this—quite often, in fact—and it's not because we're getting old and addle-brained. It's actually something that our brains are hard-wired to do! Research from the University of Notre Dame in Indiana, published in *Quarterly Journal of Experimental Psychology*, demonstrates the connection between forgetfulness and walking through doorways.

Doorways Drain Memory

This study confirms in a "real world" environment what previous research identified in a virtual environment—a phenomenon dubbed the "location-updating effect," showing that the simple act of passing through a doorway as you move from one room to another raises the likelihood that you'll forget what you were just thinking about.

The experiment: A set of volunteers (28 women and 32 men) were split into groups. Group A walked through a series of three rooms. In the first room, they were asked to place six objects (each a different shape and color) into a box and then cover it up and bring it to the next room. In the second room, after they had gone through a doorway, they were given a computer quiz, asking which objects they had put into the box just a few minutes earlier. Group B did the same thing, except they didn't walk through a series of rooms, they walked to different spots within the same room—in other words, they didn't encounter any doorways. The results? Group A—the one that walked through doorways—made 5% more errors on the memory test than Group B.

Boost Your Memory

Now, what does this act of walking through doorways mean to our brains? It is an "event boundary" that signals to your brain that your situation has changed. To understand this, think of your mind as being like a filing cabinet. When something changes—whether in time or setting—your brain acknowledges the shift by creating an "event file" as a way of keeping track of your life (without which it would be a mess!). Walking through a doorway is a signal to your brain to put what you were just thinking about into its own file…which makes information from before the location change not quite as readily available to you as it was earlier. Unfortunately, another experiment that was part of the same study showed that walking back into the original room that you were in doesn't trigger recall.

We should think of this location-updating effect as being beneficial. By creating event boundaries when entering a new space, our minds are getting refreshed, so we're able to focus on the new environment. That's helpful, when your doctor walks through the door to see you, know that she is no longer thinking about the patient that she just saw!

How can we use this information to improve our memory? One idea is to plan around it by leaving sticky notepads in every room—that way, if an idea comes to you, you can write it down immediately so you don't forget it. Another idea is to always have your smartphone handy so that you can leave yourself a voicemail or send yourself an e-mail or text. And the next time you walk purposefully into a room and instantly forget what brought you there, don't fret. It's probably nothing more than your brain's overly efficient reset button trying to get you ready for what's coming next.

Sharpen Your Memory with Music

Galina Mindlin, MD, PhD, an assistant clinical professor of psychiatry at Columbia University College of Physicians and Surgeons, supervising attending physician in the department of psychiatry and behavioral health at St. Luke's-Roosevelt Hospital Center, and clinical and executive director of the Brain Music Therapy Center, all in New York City. Dr. Mindlin is coauthor of *Your Playlist Can Change Your Life: 10 Proven Ways Your Favorite Music Can Revolutionize Your Health, Memory, Organization, Alertness, and More.* BrainMusicTreatment.com

Imagine yourself giving a toast, making a speech or delivering a big presentation at work—only to forget midway through what you wanted to say. If the mere thought makes you cringe, you'll be intrigued by a book that reveals how to use music to improve your recall. The best part is that whatever type of music appeals most to you is what will be most effective—so you don't have to suffer through music you find boring or annoying.

Because music permeates all areas of the brain, it has a tremendous capacity to deposit any memories you attach to it in assorted locations. This embeds them deeper into your brain and makes it possible to retrieve them from multiple memory banks.

You may remember the buzz back in the 1990s when a small study reported that listening to a Mozart piano sonata produced a temporary improvement in spatial reasoning skills. These modest findings were blown out of proportion in the popular press, which disseminated the exaggerated idea that "Mozart makes you smart." Subsequent research has shown that music can indeed have cognitive benefits, but it's not about Mozart. In fact, my method works with any type of music—country, classical, reggae, rock, rap, pop, opera or whatever—provided you enjoy it. The more you like the music, the more it activates brain networks and functions that amplify and sustain the effects you are working toward, such as increased concentration and alertness.

Unclutter Your Mind, Help Your Memory

Researchers from Concordia University in Montreal, Canada, have found that memory loss in older adults is not due to loss of brain function, but rather to the clutter of irrelevant information. To clear out mind clutter, try deep breathing to reduce stressors and mindfulness to bring your full attention to what you're doing.

Karen Li, et al., "The Role of Age and Inhibitory Efficiency in Working Memory Processing and Storage Components," *The Quarterly Journal of Experimental Psychology* (2010).

Choosing Your Music

So, getting back to memorizing that toast, speech or presentation, here's what you do. *First, create three lists of musical selections…*

1. Calming songs. On this list, include songs that you know from experience make you feel relaxed and balanced because they are associated with pleasurable, peaceful events from your past. For instance, one song might remind you of a blissful solitary stroll in the woods…another might bring back memories of a glorious sunset sail.

Tip: Research shows that songs with a slower tempo of 100 beats per minute (BPM) or less tend to bring on relaxation and calm.

Examples: "New York, New York" sung by Frank Sinatra or "American Pie" by Don McLean.

2. Fast-paced "activating" songs. Activating songs are mentally energizing. They might remind you of a time when you zoomed through a challenging task, celebrated an accomplishment or won a race. Generally, songs that work well in this category have a tempo of 130 BPM or faster—for instance, "Beat It" by Michael Jackson or "Jailhouse Rock" sung by Elvis Presley. Such rhythms tend to boost motivation and endurance.

3. Medium-paced activating songs. Here, select songs that recharge your batteries yet have a slightly slower tempo, typically 100 to 130 BPM. Examples include "Stayin' Alive" by the Bee Gees or the Beatles' "Lady Madonna." These types of songs help your brain lock in whatever you're trying to commit to memory.

Choose half a dozen or more selections for each list.

Reason: Feelings shift from day to day. For example, you might normally feel relaxed by a song you and your husband slow-danced to at your wedding—but if you two just had an argument, that song might upset you today. Assess your current emotions each time you use your playlists, selecting the songs that feel appropriate for the particular moment.

Once you've selected your songs, create your three playlists on your cell phone or record the songs onto CDs or cassettes.

Putting Your Playlists to Work

Now you're ready to use your music to enhance your ability to memorize whatever it is that you want to commit to memory. *Follow these steps in order…*

• **Listen to one or more calming songs to prepare your brain to be receptive to learning.** As you listen, recall as vividly as possible the relaxing, positive memories associated with each song. Continue listening until you reach that state of relaxed mental alertness.

• **Play fast-paced activating songs to shift your brain into remembering mode.** Again, as you listen, visualize in detail the upbeat memories linked with that music. Continue listening until you feel energized and ready to approach your task.

• **Turn the music off and focus on what you want to remember.** For instance, read your speech aloud from start to finish, moving around or gesturing as you read—the sound of your voice and your physical movements provide additional anchors that help cement the speech in your memory.

• **When you finish rehearsing, listen to one or more mid-tempo activating songs.** This serves as a mental cooldown to further fix the material in your mind.

• **For maximum effect, use this technique daily.** The amount of time you spend depends on the material you're trying to remember, but generally the music portion of the activity takes about 10 to 15 minutes per session.

Key: Remember to have fun with this—it should not be a chore, but instead a source of enjoyment.

Movements That Boost Memory

Teresa Liu-Ambrose, PhD, PT, associate professor, Canada Research Chair in Physical Activity, Mobility, and Cognitive Neuroscience, department of physical therapy, Aging, Mobility, and Cognitive Neuroscience Laboratory, University of British Columbia, and principal investigator, Centre for Hip Health and Mobility and Brain Research Centre, all in Vancouver, Canada. Her study was published in *Archives of Internal Medicine*.

You've probably seen elderly family members and friends slowly lose their memories, and you're determined to do everything that you can to stay sharp.

But if you think that keeping your brain healthy is something that's really difficult or time-consuming, then you will find the following news very exciting.

There's a trick, and it's not hard…nor is it very time-consuming.

The secret lies in strength training, according to Canadian researchers.

A Smarter Workout

They found that after six months of twice-weekly, hour-long workouts, people who performed strength training had better memory and brain function, compared with those who did moderate to brisk walking and those who did balance, stretching and relaxation movements (the control).

Over the course of the study, the control group showed no improvement on any of the following measures, but check out how much the strength-training group outperformed the aerobic group...

• **The strength-training group showed a 17% improvement in the brain's executive function,** which controls planning, organizing, strategizing and managing time and space, whereas the aerobic group improved just 2%!

•**In terms of associative memory function (the type of memory that links information together,** as in matching an acquaintance's name with his or her face), the aerobic group improved 47%. But that paled in comparison to the improvement made by those in the strength-training group—92%!

•**Brain imaging of the strength-training group members showed that three regions of their brains associated with cognitive behavior had become more active.** Members in the aerobic exercise group, however, did not see any improvements in this area.

We can only speculate as to why strength training came out on top. One reason may be physiological. For example, strength training may reduce systemic inflammation, increase growth factors that promote neuronal growth and maintain insulin sensitivity (conditions such as diabetes increase your risk for dementia). It may also be that during strength training, the exerciser must constantly monitor his or her actions, including breathing properly, counting the number of reps and sets and using correct form. Walking and balance/stretching/relaxation exercises, on the other hand, are more automatic. Since you don't have to pay attention as much while doing them, the moves put fewer demands on the brain.

Build Muscle—And Brain Power

To boost your memory and cognitive function, incorporate strength training into your workout schedule. Now, strength training shouldn't replace aerobic exercises or balance/stretching/relaxation exercises—those types of workouts are critical for other reasons, such as improving heart function and flexibility and reducing stress. Instead, strength training should be added to your routine if you don't already do it.

Six-Minute Memory Booster

Boost your memory in six minutes by simply taking a nap. Napping during the day—for as little as six minutes—brings better performance on memory exercises.

Possible reason: The act of falling asleep might trigger a neurological process that improves memory—even if actual sleep time is minimal.

Olaf Lahl, PhD, researcher, Institute of Experimental Psychology, University of Dusseldorf, Germany.

While study subjects performed strength training twice a week, an hour at a time, if that's too much of a time commitment (or if that's too much for you to handle, physically, right now), even adding smaller amounts of strength training to your routine is likely to help your brain a little. *Here's how to get started…*

1. Warm up. To prevent injury or strain, warm up for at least 10 minutes with light aerobic activity that will elevate your heart rate, such as brisk walking, jogging, biking or doing jumping jacks.

2. Build strength. To improve strength in all the major muscle groups, study subjects used dumbbells (starting with two to five pounds), weight lifting machines or body weight resistance (such as push-ups, lunges or squats, for example).

How many exercises you can handle during one workout depends on your level of fitness, so ask a trainer—it's best to start with only a few exercises and then gradually add more as you get stronger. Try performing two sets of each exercise, doing six to eight reps in each set, and resting for one minute in between sets. The trainer can advise you on correct form and provide guidance about when it's time to progress to heavier weights.

3. Cool down. As with the warm-up, slow down your heart rate with at least 10 minutes of light aerobic activity. Then, to prevent stiffness, gently stretch the muscles that you exercised.

And enjoy your brain power!

For a Better Memory, Just Make a Fist

Ruth E. Propper, PhD, associate professor, department of psychology, and director, cerebral lateralization laboratory, Montclair State University, New Jersey. Her study was published in *PLoS One*.

Do you struggle to remember your mental shopping list or forget people's names right after you're introduced? A recent study reveals a "handy" trick that can help—and all you need to be able to do is make a fist.

Background: Previous research has shown that when a person clenches his or her right fist, the frontal lobe on the left side of the brain shows increased activity. Similarly, clenching the left fist activates the right side of the brain.

There is a lot we don't know about how the brain works, but some experts believe that the left frontal lobe is important to encoding (creating) memories, while the right frontal lobe is associated with retrieving (recalling) memories.

So if hand clenching increases activity in different parts of the brain, would clenching the right hand activate the left side of the brain, where memories are encoded…and would clenching the left hand activate the right side of the brain, where memories are recalled?

To test the concept: 51 right-handed people were recruited to participate in the study. (Left-handed people already have superior memories, according to research, so they weren't included in this study.) All of the participants were shown a series of 36 random words, with each word being displayed for five seconds…then later, they were asked to write down as many of the words as they could.

Prior to reading and recalling the words, however, the participants were divided into five groups. In one group, each member was told to tightly squeeze a small rubber ball (to ensure a fist-clenching action) in his right hand for 90 seconds before seeing the words, then squeeze the ball in his left hand for 90 seconds before trying to recall the words. A second group did the opposite (left before reading, right before recalling). Two other groups used their right hands both times…or used their left hands both times. The fifth group didn't clench their fists at all—they simply cupped the ball gently in both hands.

Results: People who were able to recall the most words correctly were those who had squeezed with their right hands before trying to memorize the words and with their left hands before trying to recall the words. These people remembered almost 15% more words, on average, than the second-best performing group, which was the group that did not clench their fists at all. You don't consider a 15% improvement in memory such a big deal? Well, think of it in test-scoring terms—it could be the difference between an A and a C. Curiously, the three groups that did the "wrong" kind of clenching did even worse than the no-clenching group.

Give it a whirl: You don't need a ball. If you want to remember things better, simply clench your right hand for a minute and a half before you try to commit something to memory—a shopping list, a to-do list, a train schedule or the spot at the mall where you parked your car. Then clench your left hand for a minute and a half before you try to recall that list, train schedule or parking spot number. Just remember to clench right to learn, left to recall (ironically, the "R" and the "L" mnemonics are opposite). Careful—if you swap those, you could wind up recalling less than you would have if you had done no clenching at all.

A Simple Trick to Help You Remember

Mark McDaniel, PhD, professor of psychology at Washington University, St. Louis.

In a study of 57 adults (average age 72), participants were told to push a computer's "F1" key once while performing a series of cognitive and perceptual tasks. One group also was asked to touch the top of their heads when they pressed the key.

Result: Those who had touched their heads were much more likely to remember having hit the F1 key.

Theory: It's easier to recall having completed a habitual task if it is accompanied by some kind of motor task, such as touching your head or crossing your arms.

If you have trouble remembering whether you've completed a daily activity (such as taking pills): Try making a specific motion each time you perform the task.

Want to Boost Short-Term Memory? Watch a Funny Video

Gurinder Singh Bains, MD, PhD, assistant professor and primary research coordinator, Loma Linda University School of Allied Health Professions, Loma Linda, California. His study was published in *Alternative Therapies.*

You forget that thing that someone told you…this morning. You misplace your keys. You walk into the kitchen to do something…but once you get there, you forget what it is.

What you're experiencing is a decline in short-term memory. It starts to go down as early as your 40s…and it's perfectly normal. (Forgetting where you live or what your keys are for, that's a different story.)

But wouldn't it be great if there were something simple and easy that you could do to improve it?

There is. In fact it's so simple, it's funny.

How Red Skelton Enhances Brain Power

Watching a humorous video for 20 minutes may be all it takes to improve your ability to remember things you've just heard or read, found researchers at Loma Linda University in California. They showed 20 older men and women (average age 70) either a video of Red Skelton (the former clown who had a popular TV comedy show in the 1950s, '60s and early '70s)…or a montage from *America's Funniest Home Videos*.

None of the participants had any cognitive impairment. However, half of them (10) had diabetes, which is known to contribute to short-term memory loss. An additional 10 participants, who did not have diabetes nor cognitive impairment and were of the same age, were the control group. They did not watch the videos but instead were asked to sit silently in a quiet room.

Before and after watching funny videos… or sitting in silence…the participants took three components of a short-term-memory test. First, a researcher read aloud 15 words, and participants were then asked to say from memory as many as they could remember…

> ### Visualize to Memorize
>
> **Memory aid:** Instead of trying to remember a specific thing that you have to do—such as repaying money borrowed from a coworker—visualize a scene in which you actually are doing it.
>
> **Example:** Imagine taking the money out of your pocket or purse and handing it to the coworker at a specific location, such as the break room. Create the visualization before going to sleep—your brain will strengthen the image overnight, and you will be more likely to do the task the next day.
>
> Mark McDaniel, PhD, professor of psychology, Washington University in St. Louis.

a test of learning. The test was repeated five times. The same test was then given with a different list, and then participants were asked to remember what had been on the first list…a test of recall. Finally, participants were given a piece of paper with 50 words on it and asked to circle words that had been on the first list…a test of visual recognition. Finally, a little saliva was swabbed at five different points, including before and after—you'll see why in a moment.

Result? Laughter worked. After watching the humorous videos, the healthy adults did 39% better on the learning test, 44% better on the recall test and 13% better on the visual recognition test. Those with diabetes also saw significant improvements—a 33% boost in learning, a 48% jump in recall and a 17% gain in visual recognition. Sitting silently also seemed to benefit the control group but not nearly as much. Their gains were 24%, 20% and 8%, respectively.

How can a little mirth improve memory? That's where the saliva comes in.

The Stress Connection

Saliva contains cortisol, a stress hormone. All of the participants who watched the funny videos experienced a significant decrease in salivary cortisol levels. Stress, as the researchers already knew, suppresses the function of the brain's hippocampus, where short-term memory is pulled together. (Over time, chronic stress can even damage...and shrink...the hippocampus.) Feeling less stress and producing fewer stress hormones, the researchers speculate, is what led to better learning and memory in the video watchers.

This wonderfully simple experiment suggests a wonderfully simple way that we could all boost our short-term memory—watch humorous videos. There are literally thousands that are easily found online...but here are three good (and free) ones...

•**The hilarious well-known scene from the *I Love Lucy* TV show— when Lucy and Ethel get jobs at a candy factory.**

•**Comedienne Carol Burnett's spoof on *Gone With the Wind*.**

•**Frasier, from the TV comedy series *Frasier*, sings "Buttons and Bows."**

If you want to stretch out the experience, try these funny full-length movies—*Blazing Saddles* (1974), *Airplane!* (1980), *Raising Arizona* (1987), *A Fish Called Wanda* (1988), *Liar Liar* (1997), *There's Something About Mary* (1998), *Little Miss Sunshine* (2006), *Death at a Funeral* (2007) and *Brides-maids* (2011). For more choices, go to Bottomlineinc.com/classic-comedies-to-make-you-laugh-out-loud.

Of course, you don't have to watch a video to relax and laugh. Although it wasn't studied, it's a reasonable speculation that anything that lowers stress levels may enhance short-term memory. While this is the first research to show memory improvement, other research has shown that humor and laughter stimulate the immune system, make pain more tolerable, improve mood and even reduce markers of inflammation. That's fun with benefits.

Kirtan Kriya Meditation Boosts Mood and Memory

Andrew B. Newberg, MD, director of research at the Myrna Brind Center of Integrative Medicine at Thomas Jefferson University Hospital and Medical College, Philadelphia, and coauthor of *How God Changes Your Brain: Breakthrough Findings from a Leading Neuroscientist.* He is coauthor of a study published in *The Journal of Alternative and Complementary Medicine.*

We all shudder at the prospect of losing our memories and brain power as we get older. Those fears are well-founded. Among Americans age 65 and older, 13% show symptoms of Alzheimer's disease, such as memory loss, confusion, speech problems and personality changes...and an additional 10% to 20% have mild cognitive impairment, which can progress to Alzheimer's disease.

Sadly, such problems often are accompanied by depression, anxiety and other mood disorders that can further aggravate cognitive decline and erode quality of life.

What if you could think better and feel better, despite getting older, by investing just 12 minutes a day?

You might be tempted to jump at the chance. But actually, you wouldn't even have to jump—you'd get to sit.

The technique involves no drugs...requires no formal training...has no negative side effects...is easily done at home...and costs absolutely nothing.

Here's the secret...

Repeat After Me

The form of meditation called kirtan kriya (pronounced KEER-tun KREE-uh) involves repeating a mantra consisting of four syllables—Saa Taa Naa Maa—while doing a specific hand motion.

Don't laugh—because this really works!

The proof comes from a recent study involving seniors who already had memory loss from mild cognitive impairment or mild-to-moderate Alzheimer's disease. At the start and end of the study, all participants answered questions about their emotional states and underwent tests of their cognitive skills. They also had brain scans to measure cerebral blood flow in various areas of the brain linked to concentration, attention, decision-making, speech and emotions.

Do You Doodle?

Doodling improves memory. In a recent study, people who doodled while listening to a boring phone message remembered 29% more about the message than those who didn't doodle.

Jackie Andrade, PhD, professor, School of Psychology, Plymouth University, UK, and leader of a study published in *Applied Cognitive Psychology.*

One group of participants (the control group) was asked to listen to classical music for 12 minutes per day for eight weeks. The other group was taught kirtan kriya meditation and asked to perform it at home for 12 minutes daily for eight weeks.

Results: Among the kirtan kriya meditators, researchers found significant improvement in the areas of tension and fatigue, and lesser but still notable improvement in depression, anger and confusion...whereas among the music group, scores worsened in all these areas. The meditation group also showed improvement in cognitive function—and interestingly, these effects were accompanied by corresponding changes in cerebral blood flow. In contrast, among the music group, there were no significant changes in cognitive function or cerebral blood flow.

More research is needed to confirm these findings and shed light on just how this form of meditation helps with age-related memory loss and mood problems. But in the meantime, there's certainly no harm in giving it a try to see if it helps you.

How to Do Kirtan Kriya

Sit with your eyes closed. You will be using the tip of the thumb of each hand to touch the tip of each finger in sequence. As you say Saa, touch the thumb to the index finger...as you say Taa, touch the middle finger...as you say Naa, touch the ring finger...as you say Maa, touch the pinky finger. Repeat the mantra in your normal voice for two minutes...in a whisper for two minutes...silently in your head for four minutes...in a whisper again for two minutes...and in your normal voice again for two minutes.

Are you musical? Instead of speaking (or thinking) the four syllables in a monotone, you can try chanting them in a singsong fashion, hitting the note A (on Saa)...then G (on Taa)...then F (on Naa)...and then G again (on Maa).

Phone a Friend, Boost Brain Power

Oscar Ybarra, PhD, psychologist, University of Michigan Institute for Social Research, Ann Arbor, and lead author of a study of 3,610 people, published in *Personality and Social Psychology Bulletin*.

Chatting for 10 minutes a day benefits your brain as much as doing the daily crossword puzzle.

Recent finding: Social interaction—such as talking on the phone and getting together with friends—boosts memory and mental performance as effectively as more traditional kinds of mental exercise, such as word and number puzzles.

Four Easy Tricks to Remember Names Better

Scott Hagwood, author of *Memory Power* and four-time National Memory Champion. He is based in Fayetteville, North Carolina.

Imagine this—you're at a party when someone greets you by name with a hearty handshake, but you suddenly draw a blank and can't for the life of you remember his name.

How embarrassing!

We've all been in situations like that before, but we don't have to be in them again.

Your ability to remember is not necessarily something you're born with—you can train yourself to become better.

Here are my four favorite mental exercises that will train your brain to remember names more easily—and, better yet, they're all so simple!

When You Meet Someone New

Try at least one of the following tricks every time you meet a new person.

•**Alliterate to learn.** It's amazing how much memory power you can get by using alliteration, the stringing together of words that start with the same sound. To do this, when you first learn someone's name, think of a characteristic that describes this person and that starts with the first letter of the person's first name. For example, you might think to yourself, Hannah wears high heels...Tom is tall...or Donna loves drama.

•**Rhyme to remember.** Rhyming is also a powerful memory booster. So in your mind, rhyme a new person's first name with an associative characteristic. For instance, Anna eats a banana…Max plays the sax…Jim likes to swim. (This won't work for every person, of course, but it's worth trying whenever possible.)

•**Link new acquaintances with old ones.** Say you were just introduced to someone named George who seems to be a bit of a joker. Can you think of someone else you know well who is also named George and who has a similarly playful personality? If so, make a point of linking these two people in your mind ("the two jokers") so that the next time you see this new person, an image of the old George will pop into your mind—along with the name George. (Or maybe your old George has no sense of humor at all, so you can remember this "new George" as his complete opposite.)

•**Repeat the new name.** To firmly imprint a new name on your mind, repeat it both out loud and to yourself several times. Make a point of saying something such as "Great to meet you, Jason" at the beginning of the conversation and "Hope to see you again soon, Jason" at the end of the conversation.

When You Meet Someone Again

When someone you've already met reappears and his name slips your mind… what do you do? First, think of the above tricks that you used to remember this person's name in the first place. Does he have some characteristic that you notice that starts with the first letter of his name? Does he enjoy doing something that rhymes with his first name? Is he exactly like—or the complete opposite of—someone who you know who shares the same name?

If none of those methods works, don't panic. When you're in a group, be attentive, because someone else might say the name. Or just keep talking to the person without guessing at his name, because sometimes your subconscious works while you're talking, and after a few minutes, the name might come to you. If all else fails, accept defeat and politely say, "I remember talking to you before, but I've met so many people. Can you please give me your name again?" It won't be held against you!

CHAPTER 9

Sleep Well for a Healthy Brain

How Sleep Sweeps Toxins from Your Brain

Maiken Nedergaard, MD, professor of neurosurgery, codirector, Center for Translational Neuromedicine, University of Rochester Medical Center, Rochester, New York. Her research was published in *Science*.

I t's tempting to shortchange ourselves on sleep. There's so much that needs to get done while we're awake, and science has never given us a good explanation for why we sleep away one-third of our lives…until now.

Using state-of-the-art imaging technology, researchers have made a startling discovery about the purpose of sleep. It turns out that, as our bodies rest, our brains are busy sweeping away a certain type of toxic detritus that collects during the day—the same type of detritus that's linked to Alzheimer's disease and other neurodegenerative disorders. This cleanup process involves changes in the actual cellular structure of the brain—changes we can liken, oddly enough, to a busy movie theater!

Here's the latest advice on how to keep your brain in top form, plus lots of tips on how to sleep better…

Cleaning a Crowded Space

To understand this research, it helps to think of a movie theater. When a film is showing and the theater is packed, candy wrappers and popcorn and other garbage all fall to the floor. Moviegoers are making a mess, but it would be impossible to clean up while the people are still in their seats. The theater patrons wouldn't be able to concentrate on the movie…and there wouldn't be enough room for cleaners to maneuver.

Later, though, after the movie, the people clear out and the seats fold up, and there is much more room. It's easier to get to the floor beneath to sweep away all the crud that the people left behind.

Researchers from the University of Rochester Medical Center discovered that brains are like movie theaters. When we're awake, our brains are very active, guiding all our functions. As part of that process, our brains discard toxic proteins (such as the beta amyloid that's linked to Alzheimer's) and other by-products—and there's little opportunity to clean up that debris. However, as the detritus builds up, our brains can't function as well.

Cool revelation: When we sleep, our brain cells literally shrink—similar to how theater seats fold up—thus enlarging the spaces around the cells. This allows brain fluids to flow more freely, doing their job of picking up the garbage that accumulated during the day and carrying it away.

How This Discovery Was Made

In most of the human body, the lymphatic system is responsible for collecting and disposing of waste. But the lymphatic system doesn't make it past the protective blood-brain barrier that closely guards what enters the brain. Instead, cerebrospinal fluid circulates through the brain, picking up the interstitial fluid (fluid between the cells) along with the discarded proteins. This exchange of fluid was named the glymphatic system by the same Rochester researchers after they discovered the intricate network.

For the recent study, the researchers used a technique called two-photon imaging and different colored dyes to measure the rate of cerebrospinal fluid flowing through the brains of mice (the mouse brain is remarkably similar to the human brain) when the animals were awake…when they were sleeping naturally…and when they were under general anesthesia.

What the researchers found: The glymphatic system was nearly 10 times more active when the mice were asleep or anesthetized than when they were awake…and the sleeping brains removed significantly more beta amyloid and other debris. This occurred because, when the mice were asleep or anesthetized, their brain cells contracted by more than 60%, creating more space between the cells.

We already know that sufficient sleep helps us think more clearly, do better on tests, make smarter food choices and perhaps keep blood sugar under control. Though it's too early to say that getting enough sleep helps prevent Alzheimer's and other neurodegenerative diseases, the recent study findings suggest that it might—giving us yet one more reason not to shortchange our slumber time.

Get more sleep: To give your brain the rest it needs, continue reading the articles in this chapter.

Lack of Sleep Shrinks Your Brain

Study by researchers at University of Oslo, Norway, titled "Poor sleep quality is associated with increased cortical atrophy in community-dwelling adults," published in *Neurology*.

As kids we wanted no part of it. As adults we often can't get enough of it. And some of us are even proud that we "don't need" much of it. Sleep. No matter what our age or feelings about sleep, the benefits have been proven in study after study. If you don't sleep enough, even if you don't think you are tired the next day, you won't function at full capacity and you'll be more prone to making mistakes and losing focus. But now, we have learned that the penalty for not getting enough restful sleep is much worse than that.

Not getting enough sleep can literally shrink key parts of your brain.

Brain Loss Is Real

This powerful study, analyzed the brains and sleeping habits of 147 adults who ranged in age from 20 to 84. As part of the study, researchers took two MRI scans of the participants' brains three-and-a-half years apart. The participants also filled out sleep-quality questionnaires that measured how long and how well they slept over a one-month period. "Poor sleep" generally means that a person takes a long time to fall asleep and/or wakes up frequently during the night and/or doesn't get enough deep sleep.

After analyzing all the data, the researchers found that poor sleep was associated with reduced volume in the right frontal lobe of the brain. Among other things, the frontal lobe is responsible for problem-solving, making choices and memory. Poor sleep was also associated with deterioration of parts of the temporal and parietal lobes. The temporal lobe helps us sense sights and sounds but also regulates our personality, moods and behavior. The parietal lobe helps us interpret sensory information, including touch and visual perspective.

The Sleep (and Age) Connection

Sleep gives the brain the chance to repair itself in a way similar to how a "defrag" application removes noise and waste from a computer so that it runs more efficiently. But this process seems to naturally become less efficient as we age. Numerous studies have borne this out, and the study on sleep and changes to brain structure did show that changes were more conspicuous in participants who were older than 60. This led the study researchers to question whether poor sleep leads to brain changes (shrinkage and deterioration)...or, in contrast, age-related brain changes lead to poor sleep.

Sleep problems and age-related brain changes might go together as a vicious cycle. Other studies have linked poor sleep with poor cognition and an increased risk of Alzheimer's disease. But whether lack of sleep ages the brain or an aging brain thwarts sleep, there is only one side of that equation that you can profoundly alter.

This is why it is vitally important that you do everything you can to keep your brain fit. And that includes getting a restful night's sleep. *The National Sleep Foundation provides these tips...*

•**Stay on schedule.** To the extent you can, stick to the same bedtime and wake-up time to train your body to keep with a healthful sleep-wake cycle.

•**Get ready.** Relax before you go to sleep. In particular, turn off your electronic devices, such as your computer and television, about an hour before bed and let quiet time replace distraction time.

•**Skip the cat nap.** Just as snacking can ruin your appetite for mealtime, napping can leave you sleepless at night, so make an effort to limit daytime naps and, as mentioned above, reinforce a sleep- and wake-time schedule.

•**Don't force the issue.** If you can't sleep, don't force it. Get up, read a book, have a cup of soothing chamomile or passionflower tea and try again later.

•**Pass on the nightcap.** Don't drink alcohol close to bedtime. Although an alcoholic drink can help lull you to sleep, it can adversely affect how well you sleep, and you will often find yourself waking up feeling restless and dehydrated a few hours later.

More Bad News for Poor Sleepers

Older people who sleep poorly are more likely to have damaged blood vessels in the brain.

Recent study: Special sensors were used to detect nighttime awakenings in older people. Those with the greater number of arousals were 27% more likely to have hardened blood vessels and 31% more likely to have oxygen-starved tissue in the brain. These factors increase the risk for stroke and cognitive impairment.

Andrew Lim, MD, assistant professor of neurology at University of Toronto, Canada.

Is Your Bedroom Dark Enough?

Meir H. Kryger, MD, the former director of sleep medicine research and education at Gaylord Sleep Medicine of Gaylord Hospital in Wallingford, Connecticut. He is author of *A Woman's Guide to Sleep Disorders*, and has been researching and treating women's sleep problems for nearly 30 years.

Excess light at night inhibits melatonin production, which can wreak havoc with your sleep-wake cycle. This can be particularly problematic for women, given that they are already twice as likely as men to suffer from insomnia.

What's more: Melatonin also plays a role in regulating blood pressure and blood glucose levels—making it even more important to keep your bedroom sufficiently dark.

How dark is dark enough? You should not be able to see details in your room at night even after your eyes habituate to the darkness, Dr. Kryger said. If your room is too bright…

●**Get light-blocking window blinds or shades,** if necessary, to keep out streetlights and other ambient light…or at least wear a sleep mask.

●**Keep the hall light off.** If other household members are still awake when you go to bed, shut your door.

●**Replace your illuminated alarm clock.** Choose one with a built-in feature that automatically dims the clock face at night or that illuminates only when you press a button. You might even try getting rid of your alarm clock! While this seems like a shocking proposal to those who fear that they'll sleep in until noon, most people do not actually need an alarm clock because they wake up before it goes off.

●**Turn off the tube.** If you or your partner cannot get to sleep unless the television is on, there's help. A psychologist trained in cognitive behavioral therapy can retrain a person to fall asleep without the television.

Alternative: Invest in a television with a built-in timer that turns itself off and program it to do so at a time after which you would typically be asleep.

●**Check for other sources of light.** Lie in your bed and look around. Is light coming from a computer, house phone, cell phone, cable box, alarm key-

---

This Color Helps You Sleep

People who slept in blue rooms got more sleep—an average of seven hours and 52 minutes a night—than people who slept in rooms of any other color.

Possible reason: The color blue is associated with calmness and is thought to help reduce blood pressure and heart rate.

Study of 2,000 bedrooms in the UK by Travelodge, Parsippany, New Jersey. Travelodge.com

pad or any other device? Unplug it, block its glow or move the device to another room. If you need a night-light to find your way to the bathroom safely, be sure to use one that is very dim (try an energy-efficient LED night-light) and place it where its slight illumination will not disturb your slumber.

Fall Asleep Faster...Without Drugs

John Hibbs, ND, senior clinical faculty member at Bastyr University in Kenmore, Washington, and family practitioner at Bastyr Center for Natural Health, in Seattle.

I f you often toss and turn for 30 to 60 minutes or more before finally falling asleep, you may be tempted to use prescription sleeping pills.

The problem is, these make it even harder to reconnect with your normal sleep cycle, robbing you of the most restorative type of sleep.

Try natural strategies that support normal sleep patterns...

•**Go to bed earlier.** This may seem counterintuitive, as if you would only lie awake even longer than you already do. But for many people, the body's biochemically preprogrammed bedtime falls between 9:00 pm and 10:00 pm. If you stay up until midnight, your body may secrete stress hormones to cope with the demands of being awake when it wants to be asleep—and this interferes with your body clock.

Best: Move up your bedtime by an hour...give yourself several weeks to adjust...then advance your bedtime again until you're regularly hitting the hay before 10:00 pm.

•**Exercise at the right time.** Don't try to exhaust yourself with strenuous workouts, especially in the evening—this raises adrenaline levels and makes sleep more elusive.

Instead: Exercise for at least 30 minutes every morning. This reduces the stress hormone cortisol, helping to reset your biochemical clock.

•**Get wet.** Hydrotherapy—especially close to bedtime—calms the nervous system by acting on sensory receptors in the skin. Typically it is most effective to take a half-hour bath in water that's the same temperature as the skin. However, some people respond better to a hot bath...others feel more relaxed after a "contrast shower," first using hot water, then cold.

•**Adopt a pro-sleep diet.** Eliminate all stimulant foods (caffeine, sweets, monosodium glutamate) from your diet. Magnesium calms the nervous system, so eat more magnesium-rich foods (pumpkin seeds, salmon, spinach)...

and/or take 200 mg to 300 mg of supplemental magnesium twice daily. Do not skip meals—when hungry, the body secretes stress hormones that can interfere with sleep. Avoid eating too close to bedtime—a full stomach distracts the body from normal sleep physiology.

• **Try nutraceuticals.** Certain supplements help balance brain chemicals.

Recommended: At bedtime, take 500 milligrams (mg) to 1,000 mg of gamma-aminobutyric acid (GABA), a calming brain chemical. Another option is to take a bedtime dose of 50 mg to 100 mg of 5-hydroxytryptophan (5-HTP), a natural compound that relaxes by balancing levels of the brain chemical serotonin. GABA and 5-HTP can be used separately or together for as long as needed. Both are sold in health-food stores and rarely have side effects at these doses.

Better Sleep Habits

Patrick H. Finan, PhD, assistant professor of psychiatry and behavioral sciences, The Johns Hopkins University School of Medicine, Baltimore.

A late bedtime is actually better than a full night of sleep with interruptions.

Recent study: Adults who had a delayed bedtime experienced only a 12% reduction in positive mood versus 31% in those who were awakened several times during the night.

Explanation: The interrupted sleepers had less slow-wave sleep, the type that leaves you feeling restored and rested.

Can't Sleep? Surprising Causes of Insomnia

Andrew L. Rubman, ND, founder and medical director, Southbury Clinic for Traditional Medicines, Southbury, Connecticut. SouthburyClinic.com

Every night, millions of Americans have trouble falling asleep or staying asleep. Quite often this is caused by stress, anxiety, caffeine or overstimulation before bed. But there is another common cause that few people even know to consider—a nutritional deficiency of one kind or another. If you have such a deficiency, once it is identified you can easily correct it—and start enjoying peaceful slumber once again.

This is a far superior approach to prescription sleeping pills, which not only fail to address the underlying reason for sleeplessness but often are also addictive and have side effects such as disorientation and next-day fatigue.

One example: Kathryn was usually bubbly and energetic. She suddenly started dragging at work, even nodding off during meetings. At night she would awake with unpleasant and uncontrollable urges to move her legs. The surprising cause turned out to be related to Kathryn's new vegetarian diet, which she had started several months before—without meat, her diet no longer included the iron she needed. As a result, she had developed restless legs syndrome, which makes sleeping a real challenge.

The simple solution: Her doctor prescribed iron supplements and began monitoring her levels. Now Kathryn sleeps like a baby and is once again bursting with energy at the office.

Nutritional Deficiencies Interfere with Sleep

Iron and restless leg syndrome is just one of the hidden dietary deficiencies affecting sleep. If you suffer from insomnia, consult a doctor who is knowledgeable about nutritional biochemistry to assess your nutrient levels and offer diet advice and/or supplements to support your body's natural sleep processes.

The following nutrients are strongly related to sleep...

•**Calcium—nature's sedative.** When you run short on calcium, you are apt to toss and turn and experience frequent awakenings in the night. This mineral has a natural calming effect on the nervous system. It works by helping your body convert tryptophan—an essential amino acid found in foods such as turkey and eggs—into the neurotransmitter serotonin, which modulates mood and sleep. Serotonin, in turn, is converted into melatonin, a hormone that helps regulate the sleep cycle.

Advice: It's always better to get the nutrients you need from food rather than supplements. Milk and dairy products are the most common dietary sources of calcium, but many people have trouble digesting cow's milk, especially as they grow older. Excellent nondairy sources of calcium are leafy green vegetables such as kale and collard greens, canned sardines, sesame seeds and almonds. The Recommended Dietary Allowance (RDA) for adults over age 18 is 1,000 to 1,200 mg/day. For those not getting enough from dietary sources, a calcium-magnesium supplement can be effective. Take it half an hour before going to bed.

•**Relieve leg cramps with magnesium.** Nighttime leg cramps, often due to a magnesium deficiency, are a common cause of sleeplessness. Magnesium helps your body's cells absorb and use calcium, so this mineral pair works hand in hand to relax muscles, relieve painful cramps or spasms and bring on restful slumber.

Advice: Leafy green vegetables are the best source of dietary magnesium, followed by artichokes, nuts, legumes, seeds, whole grains (especially buckwheat, cornmeal and whole wheat) and soy products. A combination calcium-magnesium supplement can help this problem too. (The RDA for magnesium for adults is 400 mg/day for men and 310 mg/day for women.)

•**Vitamin B-12 for serotonin production.** Vitamin B-12 supports the production of neurotransmitters that affect brain function and sleep, helping to metabolize calcium and magnesium and working with them to convert tryptophan into the neurotransmitter serotonin. Insufficient B-12 may be a factor if you have trouble falling or staying asleep.

Advice: Foods rich in vitamin B-12 include liver and other organ meats, eggs, fish and, to a lesser degree, leafy green vegetables. For B-12 deficiency, B-12 tablets taken sublingually (dissolved under the tongue) one hour before bedtime is often effective. It's important to take a multivitamin that contains B vitamins twice daily as well, since it helps your body use the B-12 efficiently.

Note: Most B multivitamins contain B-12 but only a minimal dose, so further supplementation is usually necessary.

•**Vitamin D modulates circadian rhythms.** Again with the vitamin D! We can't hear enough about the importance of this vital nutrient, it seems—and indeed, vitamin D turns out to be essential to support your body's uptake and usage of calcium and magnesium. Its role in sleep involves modulating your circadian rhythm (the sleep/wake cycle that regulates your 24-hour biological clock).

Advice: Most Americans have less than optimal levels of vitamin D, so daily supplements of D-3, the form most efficiently used by the body, are often prescribed. Ten to 20 minutes of sunshine daily helps your body manufacture vitamin D, and foods such as fish and fortified milk are rich in this nutrient.

•**Herbs—some help, some interfere with sleep.** Although they do not specifically address nutritional deficiencies, relaxing herbal supplements such as chamomile, hops or valerian can gently nudge you toward sleep. Try them in teas, capsules or tinctures from reputable manufacturers such as Eclectic (EclecticHerb.com), taken half an hour before retiring.

Though many people swear by melatonin, there is not enough scientific evidence yet to demonstrate that this popular sleep supplement works efficiently and without long-term ill effects.

It's also important to be aware that a number of supplements are stimulating and may cause sleep irregularities in some individuals.

The biggest stimulators: Ginseng, ginkgo, St. John's wort, alpha lipoic acid and SAM-e. If you take any of these, do so early in the day, take the lowest dose that seems effective for you or discuss alternatives with your physician. These are all best used under professional guidance.

A Soothing Bedtime Snack

My favorite sleep inducer is to head upstairs each evening with a soothing bedtime beverage—either a cup of herbal tea with honey or a glass of warm milk (though not everyone's digestive system easily tolerates milk). Late-night snacking can disturb sleep, but if you must have something, keep it light. A high-protein, low-glycemic snack, such as a banana with peanut butter or half a turkey sandwich on whole-grain bread, can help encourage serotonin production... and sweet dreams.

It's 3 am and You're Awake...Again!

Michael Breus, PhD, a Scottsdale, Arizona–based clinical psychologist who is board-certified in clinical sleep disorders. He appears regularly on national television shows, including *The Doctors* and *The Dr. Oz Show*, and is a coauthor, with Debra F. Bruce, PhD, of *The Sleep Doctor's Diet Plan: Lose Weight Through Better Sleep.* TheSleepDoctor.com

In the world of sleep disorders, having difficulty staying asleep is just as troubling as having difficulty falling asleep.

Both sleep problems rob us of the consistent, high-quality rest that helps protect against high blood pressure, obesity, diabetes, stroke and depression.

Plenty of people who have nighttime awakenings turn to a prescription sleep aid, such as zolpidem (Ambien). But these pills are only a temporary fix and can cause prolonged drowsiness the next day or, in rare cases, sleepwalking or sleep-eating within hours of taking them.

A better option: Cognitive behavioral therapy for insomnia, known as CBT-I, is now recommended as a first-line treatment for chronic sleep problems.* With CBT-I, you work with a specially trained therapist (typically for six to eight sessions) to identify, challenge and change the patterns of thinking that keep you awake at night. A 2015 study found CBT-I, which is typically covered by health insurance, to be more helpful than *diazepam* (Valium), commonly used as a sleep aid, in treating insomnia.

But if you are not quite ready to commit to a course of CBT-I—or even if you do try it—there are some simple but effective strategies you can use at home to help you stay asleep and get the deep rest you need.

Best approaches to avoid nighttime awakenings…

•**Get more omega-3 fatty acids.** While the research is still preliminary, a new study published in *Sleep Medicine* found that the more omega-3–rich fatty fish adults ate, the better their sleep quality.

My advice: Eat fatty fish…and to ensure adequate levels of omega-3s, consider taking a fish oil supplement (one to two 1,000-mg capsules daily).**

•**Avoid "blue light" at night.** Exposure to blue light—the kind emitted by smartphones, computers, tablets and LED TVs—disrupts sleep patterns by blocking the release of the sleep hormone melatonin. Even if you do fall asleep fairly easily, blue light exposure may come back to haunt you in the form of a middle-of-the-night wake up.

If you can't force yourself to power down your electronics within two hours of bedtime, try positioning handheld devices farther away from your eyes than usual.

In addition, consider various apps that filter blue light on your smartphone or tablet. Some operating systems are automatically programmed with this feature—Apple's iOS 9.3 offers Night Shift, for example. Using your device's geolocation and clock, the colors of your display are automatically shifted to the warmer end of the spectrum (which is less disruptive to sleep) around sundown. Free apps for Android devices include Night Shift: Blue Light Filter and Twilight.

•**Use special lightbulbs.** If you wake up in the middle of the night and make a trip to the bathroom, the glare of the bathroom light tells your brain "It's morning!"

*To find a CBT-I therapist, consult the Society of Behavioral Sleep Medicine, Behavioral Sleep.org. You can also try the free CBT-i Coach app, available at iTunes or Google Play.

**Consult your doctor if you take medication.

What helps: Use low-blue lightbulbs in your bathroom and bedroom that don't block the release of melatonin. A variety are available from Lighting Science (LSGC.com). Or look online for night-lights designed to emit low levels of blue light.

If You Do Wake Up

Even if you follow the steps described above, you may still have occasional nighttime awakenings with trouble falling back asleep (meaning you are awake for at least 25 minutes).

Experiment with the following strategies to see what works best for you...

•**Resist the urge to check e-mail or do anything else on your phone.** Even short exposures to blue light are enough to suppress melatonin. Mentally stimulating activities, such as loud TV, are also best avoided. (However, a TV at low volume with the setting adjusted to dim the screen can be a great distractor for an active mind at night.)

My advice: Choose a relaxing activity like reading, listening to soothing music or knitting. If you read, use a book light or a bedside-table lamp that has one of the special bulbs mentioned earlier.

•**Don't look at the clock.** If you do, you'll start doing the mental math of how many hours you have left until you need to wake up. This will cause anxiety that will spike your levels of cortisol and adrenaline, sleep-disrupting hormones that make you feel wide awake!

My advice: Turn your clock around, and try counting backward from 300 by threes to distract yourself and promote drowsiness.

Also helpful: Try the "4-7-8 method"—inhale for four seconds...hold your breath for seven...and exhale slowly for eight. Breathe in this manner for up to 15 to 20 minutes or until you fall asleep. Inhaling and holding in air increases oxygen in the body, which means your body doesn't have to expend as much energy. The slow exhale helps you unwind and mimics the slow breathing that takes place during sleep, which will help you fall asleep.

•**Turn on some pink noise.** The well-known "white noise"—used to mask conversations and potentially startling sounds—is comprised of all frequencies detectable by the human ear. Pink noise, on the other hand, has a lower, softer frequency. Pink noise is generally considered more relaxing and has a steady sound like gentle rain.

Sleep experts believe that our brains respond better to the lower spectrum of pink noise than to the fuller spectrum of white noise. The result is a more peaceful and sleep-conducive feeling.

My advice: Search for a free app that contains pink noise, and listen to it with earphones on your smartphone, laptop or tablet if you wake up in the middle of the night. Just be sure to glance only briefly at the screen when turning on the device, and turn off the screen light while listening. You can set the pink noise to play for a set amount of time, such as 30 minutes. As an alternative, you can purchase a pink-noise generator online.

Foods That Sabotage Sleep

Bonnie Taub-Dix, RDN, CDN, a registered dietitian and director and owner of BTD Nutrition Consultants, LLC, on Long Island and in New York City. She is author of *Read It Before You Eat It.* BonnieTaubDix.com

You know that an evening coffee can leave you tossing and turning into the wee hours. *But other foods hurt sleep, too…*

•**Premium ice cream.** Brace yourself for a restless night if you indulge in Häagen-Dazs or Ben & Jerry's late at night. The richness of these wonderful treats comes mainly from fat—16 to 17 grams of fat in half a cup of vanilla, and who eats just half a cup?

Your body digests fat more slowly than it digests proteins or carbohydrates. When you eat a high-fat food within an hour or two of bedtime, your digestion will still be "active" when you lie down—and that can disturb sleep.

Also, the combination of stomach acid, stomach contractions and a horizontal position increases the risk for reflux, the upsurge of digestive juices into the esophagus that causes heartburn—which can disturb sleep.

•**Chocolate.** Some types of chocolate can jolt you awake almost as much as a cup of coffee. Dark chocolate, in particular, has shocking amounts of caffeine.

Example: Half a bar of Dagoba Eclipse Extra Dark has 41 milligrams of caffeine, close to what you'd get in a shot of mild espresso.

Chocolate also contains theobromine, another stimulant, which is never a good choice near bedtime.

•**Beans.** Beans are one of the healthiest foods. But a helping or two of beans—or broccoli, cauliflower, cabbage or other gas-producing foods—close to bedtime can make your night, well, a little noisier than usual. No one sleeps well when suffering from gas pains. You can reduce the "backtalk" by drinking a mug of chamomile or peppermint tea at bedtime. They're carminative herbs that aid digestion and help prevent gas.

●**Spicy foods.** Spicy foods temporarily speed up your metabolism. They are associated with taking longer to fall asleep and with more time spent awake at night. This may be caused by the capsaicin found in chili peppers, which affects body temperature and disrupts sleep. Also, in some people, spicy foods can lead to sleep-disturbing gas, stomach cramps and heartburn.

Sleeping Pills Are Just Plain Dangerous

Robert Langer, MD, MPH, principal scientist and medical director, Jackson Hole Center for Preventive Medicine, Wyoming.

It's bad enough that people are so desperate for sleep that they resort to taking any of a long list of pharmaceuticals in an effort to help them get a good night's rest. Even worse is that these theoretical helpers come with a long list of associated dangers, including addiction.

Well guess what? The list of dangers just got longer.

Research, conducted by physicians at the Scripps Clinic Viterbi Family Sleep Center in San Diego and Jackson Hole Center for Preventive Medicine (JHCPM) in Wyoming, has shown that use of sleeping pills has been associated with an increased risk for cancer and death.

The most troubling part is that this study found that it's not just daily users who are at risk—those who use them less than twice a month may even be at risk.

Flower Sleep Remedy

Not sleeping well? Try lavender. When a bottle of lavender oil was left open within three feet of the bedsides of adults who were hospitalized, they slept significantly better and had lower overnight blood pressure.

Why: The soothing scent of lavender calms the nervous system.

To improve anyone's sleep: Use lavender oil in an aromatherapy diffuser at bedtime, or put a few drops on a cotton ball, and tuck it into your pillowcase.

Karen Davis, PhD, professor, department of health policy and management, The Johns Hopkins Hospital, Baltimore.

Gentle Ways to Get Better Sleep

Jamison Starbuck, ND, a naturopathic physician in family practice and a guest lecturer at the University of Montana, both in Missoula. She is a past president of the American Association of Naturopathic Physicians and a contributing editor to *The Alternative Advisor: The Complete Guide to Natural Therapies and Alternative Treatments.*

When you're really wrestling with insomnia, it's tempting to go to your doctor and ask for one of the sleep medications we see advertised on TV—Ambien or Lunesta—or an older tranquilizing drug such as Valium. While short-term use of one of these drugs might make sense for a person who feels his/her overall health is being threatened by insomnia, I generally advise against this approach. Sure, these drugs may temporarily allow you to sleep, but they don't cure insomnia. *My advice…*

• **Do some detective work.** Thinking about your own sleep issues and making some written notes can be a big help. When do you typically go to bed? How often do you have insomnia? Do you have trouble falling asleep or wake in the middle of the night? Also, look at when your problem started to determine whether it coincided with any health issues, use of new medications or habits, such as working late hours, that could lead to insomnia.

• **Get your doctor involved.** Discuss your notes with your doctor. Chronic pain, hormonal changes (including those related to hyperthyroidism and menopause) and serious illness, such as cancer and heart or lung disease, can cause insomnia. If any of these conditions is to blame, getting proper treatment may well take care of the insomnia, too.

After you've consulted your doctor, try these gentle methods…*

• **Avoid high-protein dinners.** Protein is often hard to digest. Eating a lot at dinner can lead to gastrointestinal distress that may result in insomnia. Instead, eat foods that are easy to digest (such as soup and salad) for dinner, and have larger, protein-rich meals midday.

Also helpful: Take a 2,000-mg omega-3 supplement with your evening meal. When taken before bedtime, these healthful fats can have a calming effect on the brain, promoting sleep.

• **Try Calms Forté.** This homeopathic preparation is effective and extremely safe.

*Check with your doctor before trying supplements, especially if you take medication and/or have a chronic medical condition.

Typical dose: One tablet under the tongue at bedtime and whenever you wake up in the middle of the night (up to six tablets per 24-hour period). Calms Forté, made by Hylands, is available at natural groceries and pharmacies.

•**Add skullcap.** If the steps above don't give you relief, you may want to also try this potent herb to relax the "busy brain" experience that often keeps people awake. I recommend using skullcap in tincture form—30 to 60 drops (one-sixteenth to one-eighth teaspoon) in a cup of chamomile or spearmint tea at bedtime.

Note: Skullcap can make some people too sleepy. If you are sensitive to medication, try just 10 drops of skullcap at bedtime—or simply drink chamomile or mint tea as a sedative.

•**Use melatonin with care.** If you'd rather try this popular sleep aid, do so thoughtfully. Melatonin is a hormone. Taking too much can trigger irritability. Melatonin supplements may also raise women's estrogen levels, increasing overall inflammation in the body. I recommend taking no more than 3 mg of melatonin in a 24-hour period and often start my patients on a daily dose of only 1 mg. Take melatonin 30 minutes before bedtime.

Natural Cures Tailored to Your Sleep Problem

Laurie Steelsmith, ND, LAc, a licensed naturopathic physician and acupuncturist in private practice in Honolulu and author of *Natural Choices for Women's Health*. DrSteel smith.com

Let's say you have trouble sleeping. You want to avoid prescription and even over-the-counter sleep drugs, which can be habit-forming and have bad side effects. You're leaning toward a safer, natural alternative…possibly melatonin.

You're wondering, "What's the best sleep supplement?"

But that's the wrong question.

The right question is, "What's the best supplement to help me with my specific sleep problem?"

There are lots of herbs and supplements to choose from that can help with sleep problems. Some work better for certain situations than others. In fact, melatonin, the most popular sleep supplement, is usually not the best choice (see page 208).

There are also lifestyle changes that may help with each specific situation. For most people, these lifestyle changes—and, if needed, specific herbs and supplements tailored to particular situations—can help restore good sleep.

One caveat: If you have a chronic medical condition or take any kind of medication, check with your doctor before taking supplements.

If You Have Trouble Falling Asleep

This is usually due to a busy mind, anxious thoughts and high levels of the stress hormone cortisol in the evening, when it should be low.

Before taking supplements, do this for a week: Try a calming bath to unwind at night, or relaxation therapy such as meditation or listening to a guided imagery recording. Lower the lights, quiet the house, turn off all electronics. If you're still experiencing insomnia after a week, try taking one of the following supplements to help you drop more easily into sleep…and make sure you continue with the lifestyle changes.

•**Phosphatidylserine.** This supplement, usually derived from cabbage or soy, decreases cortisol at night. Phosphatidylserine can help optimize your reaction to stress and support the proper release of cortisol. A product called Seriphos contains 90 mg of phos-

phatidylserine. Start with one pill an hour or two before bedtime taken with a small high-protein snack (such as a cracker with almond butter) for better absorption and to prevent stomach upset. If you tolerate it well and you need more support, take two pills. You can take up to two pills before bed and two in the middle of the night if you're waking up. Side effects are rare—occasion-

Nose Trick Puts You to Sleep

Do you have difficulty falling asleep? Look to your nose! The left nostril is connected to the right hemisphere of the brain. Breathing through the left nostril can activate the parasympathetic nervous system, which counteracts stress and helps calm you and put you into a sleep mode. *Here's the way to put that nostril to work to bring on the sleep you need…*

Lie on your right side, which will help open your left nostril, then use the thumb or index finger of your right hand to close the right nostril. Take long, deep breaths through your left nostril for a few minutes…and you will feel much more relaxed and closer to sleep.

Pill-Free Cure for Insomnia

If you just can't catch those Zs, try this acupressure trick. Just before you go to bed, press the center of the bottoms of your heels with your thumbs. The easiest way to do this is to lie on your back (on a carpeted floor is best) and bend your knees, using your right hand on your left foot and left hand on your right. Press as hard as you can without cramping your hands. Keep pressing for at least two minutes—up to four minutes is even better. You should feel yourself starting to really relax, with tension leaving your body. Ease into bed for blissful zzzzzzzs.

Joan Wilen and Lydia Wilen are folk-remedy experts based in New York City. They are authors of *Bottom Line's Treasury of Home Remedies & Natural Cures* and *Bottom Line's Household Magic.*

ally, you might feel a little sleepy the next day, and very rarely, a paradoxical feeling of being more awake at bedtime. Avoid phosphatidylserine if you have kidney problems.

●**Valerian root and GABA.** Valerian root (an herb) and GABA (gamma-aminobutyric acid, an amino acid supplement) help to calm the nervous system. They both bind to GABA receptors in the brain and can be taken alone or together. The standard dose of valerian root is 300 mg to 500 mg of a standardized extract of 0.5% essential oils taken one hour before bedtime. The standard dose of GABA is 250 mg to 1,000 mg taken one hour before bed. Start with GABA first to see if you get the desired effect. Start with 250 mg at night, and increase the dose to up to 1,000 mg if necessary. (GABA can cause serious cardiovascular side effects and nightmares in very large doses—10,000 mg—and should be avoided entirely by pregnant and lactating women.)

Valerian root is safe and effective for most people, but side effects can occur, such as headaches, insomnia, excitability and a feeling of uneasiness. If falling asleep is still a huge effort, take both at the same time. It's safe to take valerian root (up to 500 mg at night) and GABA (250 mg to 500 mg at night) for up to three months—while working on the underlying causes of your insomnia.

If You Have Trouble Staying Asleep

Nighttime wakening can be one of the most difficult-to-treat sleep conditions.

One lifestyle tip: Make sure you're eating adequate calories for dinner. Skipping dinner causes your blood sugar level to drop, which increases cortisol in your body and can wake you up. Eating a solid, healthful dinner that contains all three macronutrients—protein, fat and carbohydrate—can mitigate this.

●**5-HTP.** Another common culprit is too little serotonin. This neurotransmitter makes us feel happier, calmer and more balanced and plays an important role in sleep. To boost serotonin, try 5-HTP. This supplement is the active form of tryptophan, an amino acid that your body needs to make serotonin. It's often used to help people who are depressed, a condition that can be characterized by low serotonin levels. But your levels can be lower than ideal even if you aren't experiencing depression—and if so 5-HTP supplements can help you stay asleep. Start with 100 mg taken at least one hour before bed, and gradually increase to 300 mg if you need it. At these doses, side effects are rare—but don't take this supplement if you are taking a prescription antidepressant (such as an SSRI) that also increases serotonin levels.

If Menopausal Symptoms Are Waking You Up...

Women who are in the menopausal transition (perimenopause) often have sleep problems due to hormonal fluctuations.

First step: Get your hormone levels assessed to see if your estrogen is too high and progesterone too low, or if both hormones are low. If progesterone is low, chaste tree berry (see below) can balance levels, but sometimes bioidentical hormones can help, too. Start with bioidentical progesterone, and if that isn't enough, try an estrogen cream to apply to the vagina or vulva.

•**Chaste tree berry.** For women in perimenopause, this herb can help to naturally increase waning progesterone levels. Progesterone is a calming hormone and can help even out a woman's fluctuating hormonal levels through its action on the pituitary gland. It has been shown to help support healthy ovulation, which is essential for supporting progesterone levels, even during perimenopause. Try Asensia, a chaste tree berry-containing product that also contains other ingredients, including L-arginine and green tea extract, which in combination help the chaste tree berry be better utilized by your body. It is very safe to use.

•**Especially for night sweats.** Asensia can help in women who are waning in progesterone, and Seriphos works great for insomnia associated with night sweats.

•**Got to pee?** Try to get up and do your business without turning on the lights or peeking at the clock. But if every night you're being wakened about the same time, you could try taking a drop of a homeopathic sleep remedy such as Quietude by Boiron. It contains homeopathic doses of hyoscyamus niger, nux moschata, passiflora incarnata and stramonium. The tablets can be placed under the tongue and allowed to dissolve while you drift off to sleep.

If You Have Jet Lag or Work the Night Shift

If you've crossed a few time zones or regularly work through the night, you know that it throws off your circadian rhythm, making it hard to get back into a regular sleep pattern. Expose yourself to sunlight, especially morning sunlight, when you can, which will help regulate your internal clock. *A few specific tips...*

•**For jet lag,** before your trip, wake up and go to sleep earlier several days before a trip heading east...go to sleep later for a westward trip...and when you get to your destination, make yourself get up in the morning and work out.

•**For shift work,** you'll sleep better and be more awake on the job if you stick to the same sleep and wake schedule every day, even on days you're not working.

If these approaches don't work for you, consider...

•**Melatonin.** A lot of people think they should pop melatonin whenever they have trouble sleeping, but it's really only best for resetting a body clock that has been thrown off by shifting time zones or shift work. A typical dose is 3 mg under the tongue to be taken within one hour of when you want to fall asleep. For jet lag, you can use it for a few nights to settle into a new time zone...or it can be used longer by people who have night shifts. It's often used long term for men and women who change their day/night sleep cycle frequently—such as doctors and nurses. Side effects can include headache, short-term depression, daytime sleepiness, dizziness, cramps and irritability. Some people are very sensitive to melatonin, and even a typical 3-mg dose may be too much for them. Start with a 1-mg dose and slowly increase to 3 mg if you tolerate it well. This is not recommended for children or young women who want to get pregnant. Because melatonin levels tend to naturally drop as people get older, melatonin is best for people older than 50.

Nourish Your Calm

All these strategies can help you feel rested and restored, but to truly improve sleep, you need to take stock of how your energies are being spent—and adjust your lifestyle so that you nourish a calm nervous system. This alone will do wonders for people who are having trouble sleeping.

After all, you can't expect to be mentally overstimulated all day and then have your mind turn off at night like a switch. Exercise is also key—it discharges stress and tension, and encourages sound sleep. Get regular physical exercise but avoid exercising in the three hours before bedtime, when it could rev you up.

Finally...as a last resort, it's ok to occasionally take prescription sleep aides. There is a time and place for them especially for those who have intractable insomnia. Some need these only occasionally, but others stay on these long term.

Recommended: Benadryl, which allows a person to wake up, rather than others such as Ambien, which could put a person into a trancelike state where he/she doesn't remember what he has done if he gets up in the middle of the night.

Sleep Soundly: Safe, Natural Insomnia Solution

Rubin Naiman, PhD, psychologist specializing in sleep and dream medicine and clinical assistant professor of medicine at the University of Arizona's Center for Integrative Medicine. He is author of the book *Healing Night* and coauthor with Dr. Andrew Weil of the audiobook *Healthy Sleep*. DrNaiman.com

A good night's sleep…there's nothing more restorative—or elusive…for the 64% of Americans who report regularly having trouble sleeping. A disconcertingly high percentage of the sleepless (nearly 20%) solve the problem by taking sleeping pills. But sleeping pills can be dangerously addictive, physically and/or emotionally—and swallowing a pill when you want to go to sleep doesn't address the root cause of the problem. What, exactly, is keeping you up at night?

Slow Down…

Most of our sleep problems have to do not with our bodies, per se, but with our habits. The modern American lifestyle—replete with highly refined foods and caffeine-laden beverages, excessive exposure to artificial light in the evening, and "adrenaline-producing" nighttime activities, such as working until bedtime, watching TV or surfing the Web—leaves us overstimulated in the evening just when our bodies are designed to slow down…and, importantly, to literally cool down as well.

Studies show that a cooler core body temperature—and warmer hands and feet—make you sleepy. Cooling the body allows the mind and the heart to get quiet. He believes that this cooling process contributes to the release of melatonin, the hormone that helps to regulate the body's circadian rhythm of sleeping and waking.

Deep Green Sleep

My integrative approach to sleep defines healthy sleep as an interaction between a person and his/her sleep environment. I call this approach Deep Green Sleep. My goal was to explore all of the subtleties in a person's life that may be disrupting sleep. This takes into account your physiology, emotions, personal experiences, sleeping and waking patterns and your attitudes about sleep and the sleeping environment. This approach is unique because it values the subjective and personal experience of sleep, in contrast with conventional sleep treatment, which tends to rely on computer printouts of sleep studies—otherwise known as "treating the chart."

It's important to realize that lifestyle habits and attitudes are hard to change, so it often can take weeks, even months, to achieve Deep Green Sleep. The good news is that the results are lasting and may even enhance your waking life.

Here's how you can ease into the night…

•**Live a healthful waking life.** The secret of a good night's sleep is a good day's waking. This includes getting regular exercise (but not within three hours of bedtime) and eating a balanced, nutritious diet.

•**Cool down in the evening.** It's important to help your mind and body cool down, starting several hours before bedtime, by doing the following…

•**Avoid foods and drinks that sharply spike energy,** such as highly refined carbohydrates and anything with caffeine, at least eight hours before bedtime.

•**Limit alcohol in the evening**—it interferes with sleep by suppressing melatonin. It also interferes with dreaming and disrupts circadian rhythms.

•**Avoid nighttime screen-based activities within an hour of bedtime.** You may think that watching TV or surfing the Web are relaxing things to do, but in reality these activities are highly stimulating. They engage your brain and expose you to relatively bright light with a strong blue wavelength that mimics daylight and suppresses melatonin.

•**Create a sound sleeping environment.** It is also important that where you sleep be stimulation-free and conducive to rest.

In your bedroom…

•**Be sure that you have a comfortable mattress, pillow and bedding.** It's amazing how many people fail to address this basic need—often because their mattress has become worn out slowly, over time, and they haven't noticed.

•**Remove anything unessential from your bedside table that may tempt you to stay awake,** such as the TV remove control or stimulating books.

•**When you are ready to call it a night,** turn everything off—radio, TV and, of course, the light.

•**Keep the room cool (68°F or lower).**

•**Let go of waking.** Each day, allow your mind and body to surrender to sleep by engaging in quieting and relaxing activities starting about an hour before bedtime, such as…

- Gentle yoga
- Meditation
- Rhythmic breathing
- Reading poetry or other nonstimulating material
- Journaling
- Taking a hot bath

Also: Sex seems to help most people relax and can facilitate sleep, in part because climaxing triggers a powerful relaxation response.

For more information on transforming sleep and dreams, visit Dr. Naiman's website at Dr.Naiman.com.

The 15-Minute Secret to Sleeping Better (Boost Energy and Mood, Too)

Michael Terman, PhD, director of the Center for Light Treatment and Biological Rhythms at Columbia University Medical Center, New York City. He is founder and president of the Center for Environmental Therapeutics (CET), New York City. A leading authority on the circadian clock and the role that light plays in regulating it, Dr. Terman is coauthor of *Chronotherapy: Resetting Your Inner Clock to Boost Mood, Alertness, and Quality Sleep.*

Many of us have trouble sleeping and experience times during the day when our energy or mood lags. This can be more pronounced in the fall and winter when the days are shorter and darker.

The good news is that you don't have to turn to medication to fix these problems. The way to restful sleep, increased energy and a better mood may be as easy as exposing yourself to the right amount of light at the right time of day. *Here, how to do it…*

How Light Affects Us

Many of us spend most of our days indoors. Even if our homes or offices seem to get a lot of natural light through windows, a light meter held in the room would show that the amount of light indoors registers much lower than just outside the window. In the evening, when our inner clock needs to wind down, we are inundated by artificial light from lamps, computer monitors and television screens. In our bedrooms at night, a night-light, streetlights, bathroom light, etc., can disturb sleep timing and quality.

Bright-Light Therapy

By changing the amount and patterns of your daily light exposure, remarkable changes in your mood, energy and sleep can occur within days.

What to do: Buy a fluorescent light box that provides 10,000 lux of illumination (lux measures the light level reaching your eyes from the source). That is the equivalent of the amount of light that you would get while walking on the beach on a clear morning about 40 minutes after sunrise. The lamp should have a screen that filters out ultraviolet (UV) rays, which can be harmful to the eyes and skin. It should give off only white light, not colored light, which has been hyped to be especially potent but is visually disturbing and no better than white. To be sure of a big enough field of illumination, the screen area should be about 200 square inches (for example, 12 inches x 16 inches) or larger.

A good brand that meets all of the requirements is the DL930 Day-Light Classic by UpLift Technologies. It costs about $150. Many insurance companies will fully or partially cover the cost of a light box if you provide a physician's letter. Adjust the light box so that the light comes from above your line of sight and you feel comfortable and are not squinting. You should be positioned 12 to 13 inches from the screen. You can get the benefits of the light while talking on the phone, using your computer or enjoying breakfast. You sit facing forward, focused on the work surface, while the light shines down at your head from in front.

While side effects from light therapy are rare and relatively minor, they can occur. If you experience eyestrain, headache, queasiness or agitation after beginning light therapy, reduce the light dose by sitting farther away from the light box or shorten the duration of exposure.

Sleep Problems

When do you prefer to go to sleep, and when do you like to wake up? Your answer indicates your chronotype, your individual inner clock. To determine your chronotype, take the chronotherapy quiz at CET.org. Click on "Assessments," then "Automated Online Confidential Self-Assessments" and then "Your Circadian Rhythm Type (Auto MEQ)."

The quiz will tell you the amount and timing of light therapy that will work best for you, but here are general recommendations...

•**You fall asleep too early.** You find it hard to stay awake at night and typically wake up very early in the morning.

Prescription for light therapy: Use a bright-light therapy box for 15 to 30 minutes about an hour before you typically get sleepy.

Other helpful strategies for staying awake and pushing your sleep cycle forward...

- **Make lunch your major meal of the day,** then eat only a light dinner.

- **Avoid napping, especially in the afternoon and evening.** Instead, distract yourself from your fatigue by moving around and doing stretches.

- **Turn up room lights during the evening.**

- **You fall asleep too late.** You try to get to bed at a decent hour but can't fall asleep. Then you have trouble waking up for work or school.

Prescription for light therapy: Use a light box for 15 to 30 minutes within 10 minutes after your natural wake-up time. If this time is later than your work schedule allows, begin light therapy on a long weekend. Then begin shifting your wake-up time and light-therapy schedule earlier—in 15-minute increments—as soon as you feel comfortable waking up at the new time.

More strategies for shifting your inner clock earlier include...

- **Finish dinner at least three hours before bedtime.** Avoid alcohol after dinner.

- **Minimize napping,** especially in the second half of the day. Try to get outdoors, keep moving and do some stretches instead.

- **Keep your bedroom dark until you wake up.** Early morning light seeping in through the windows actually can worsen a late-sleep pattern.

- **You sleep fitfully.**

Prescription for light therapy: Take light therapy—or spend time in the sun—in the middle of the day. Enhancing midday light exposure often improves sleep quality at night.

Other strategies to help you sleep through the night include...

- **Do not drink alcohol after dinner.**

- **Keep your bedroom dark.**

If you tend to wake up at night to use the bathroom, install amber-colored night-lights in the bathroom and hallway instead of turning on bright lights, which can disrupt your sleep.

•**You are unable to fall back to sleep after waking in the middle of the night.** There could be many causes for this type of sleep problem, such as anxiety, depression and physical illness, so it is best to consult a doctor. However, using light therapy in the evening to push sleep onset later (see "fall asleep too early") may help some people sleep through the night.

Energy and Mood

You can use bright-light therapy at any time during the day to increase your energy and alertness. Some people can quickly recharge with a brief session of light therapy (as little as 10 minutes) when they first feel an energy slump.

Caution: See a doctor if you are chronically lethargic—this can be a sign of depression, a medical sleep disorder (such as apnea) or other illness.

If you're feeling sad or mildly depressed, the light-therapy regimen is the same as the prescription for falling asleep too late.

Caution: It can be difficult for an individual to know the difference between mild depression and moderate or severe depression. If you are suffering from moderate or severe depression, a physician will need to monitor your progress with light therapy and consider other treatment options. To help determine where you fall on the depression spectrum, go to CET.org.

Mindfulness Brings on the ZZZs

David S. Black, PhD, MPH, assistant professor of preventive medicine at Keck School of Medicine, University of Southern California, Los Angeles, and leader of a study published in *JAMA Internal Medicine.*

Mindfulness meditation can help sleep. People over age 55 with sleep problems who were taught a standardized, structured course of meditation reported significantly better sleep quality. You can learn this meditation through programs such as Mindful Awareness Practices or Mindfulness-Based Stress Reduction.

To Get to Sleep Fast, Do These 6 Easy Yoga Moves

Loren Fishman, MD, assistant clinical professor of rehabilitation and regenerative medicine, Columbia Medical School, New York City, medical director, Manhattan Physical Medicine and Rehabilitation, and author of several books on yoga for health, including the upcoming book, *Healing Yoga: Proven Postures to Treat Twenty Common Ailments—from Backache to Bone Loss, Shoulder Pain to Bunions, and More.*

Losing a good night's sleep is a bummer, isn't it? You walk around in a groggy fog the next day and run the risk of getting snippy with co-workers, friends and loved ones because sleep deprivation has made you grumpy. So many factors in modern daily life can make it tough for us to fall asleep, stay asleep and rest peacefully. Gentle stretching and certain breathing techniques, such as long deep breathing, are good to do right before bedtime. You can also de-stress and set the stage for a good night's sleep with a quick set of simple yoga poses.

Yoga is a powerful tool to relieve stress and help your body relax and prepare for sleep. By stretching muscles, yoga poses trigger mechanisms in the body that send powerful relaxing signals to the brain. When performed daily, yoga can make us into better sleepers.

Try the following yoga routine nightly at bedtime. Poses can even be done while in bed. Otherwise, do them on a cushioned surface on the floor. A plush blanket or towel will do if you don't have carpeting or a yoga mat.

•**Seated forward bend.** This will give a great stretch to your legs and back muscles. To prepare for the forward bend, sit with your legs straight in front of you. First, stretch one leg and then the other by extending from the hip through the heel to elongate the leg. Then relax your legs and stretch your arms straight upward to feel your torso and back extend long and lean. Now you are ready to bend forward from the hips and reach out with your hands to grasp your ankles or feet (or 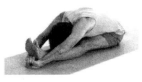 as far down your legs as you comfortably can—you should be stretching, but not straining). Let gentle, deep breaths help you relax into the stretch. Hold this pose for one to three minutes.

•**Revolved abdomen pose.** This pose massages the abdominal organs, gives a nice stretch to the lower back and muscles across the rib cage and opens the chest so you can breathe more deeply. To do it, lie on your back, bend your knees to your chest and stretch your arms out to your sides. With bent knees pressed together, inhale. Then, while exhaling, twist from your hips to lower your legs to the right while turning your face to the left. Again, give yourself 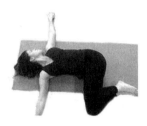 a nice stretch, but do not strain or force yourself to go deeper into the pose than you comfortably can. Hold the pose for five breaths, then bring your knees and head back to center. Repeat the pose on the opposite side by dropping your knees to the left while turning your head to the right. Hold the pose for five breaths.

•**Reclining big toe pose.** This is a leg lift that gives a good stretch to the muscles all down the back of the leg. Unless you are very limber, you will need a prop to help you get the most stretch. The prop can be a long belt, scarf, cord or necktie that you can brace against the arch or ball of your foot and use as a lever to stretch your leg until your foot faces the ceiling. To do this posture, lie on your back, take a deep breath, and, while gently exhaling, bend your right knee to your chest and loop the prop around the arch or ball of the right foot, 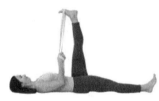 holding the ends of the prop in both hands. Inhale while straightening your knee so that your right heel is turned toward the ceiling. Guide the prop to comfortably increase the stretch. Hold this pose for a minute or two and then repeat with the other leg.

•**Child's pose.** This restorative yoga pose helps get more blood flowing in the head and can be so deeply relaxing that when you roll out of it, you may just nod off to sleep like a baby. Begin by kneeling so that you are sitting on your heels, and take a nice, deep, relaxing breath. Bend forward while exhaling and place your forehead on the floor (or on your bed if that's where you are doing the exercise). Place your arms at your sides so that the hands, palms turned up, are near your feet. As you breathe, especially focus on relaxing your back and shoulders. Hold this pose for five to seven long, slow deep breaths.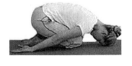

•**"Stop-action" breathing.** This is an easy and deeply relaxing breathing technique that strengthens the respiratory system. While lying down on your back in bed, exhale completely through the nose. Then inhale a little bit of air—just enough for a count of two or three seconds. Hold that little bit of breath for two or three seconds and, without exhaling, take another two or three seconds of breath, hold, and keep on taking those little sips of air, inhaling and pausing, until your lungs are full as if you've just taken only one big breath instead of a series of small ones. Hold for a second or two. Then slowly exhale in the same manner, exhaling a little bit for two or three seconds, pausing with breath held for two or three seconds and continuing like this until you've completely exhaled air from the lungs. Do four or five rounds of this breathing technique, taking a normal breath between each round of the stop-action breaths.

•**Corpse pose.** If you're not in your bed yet, it's time to crawl into it and get into this pose—you're going to be asleep soon! Lie on your back with your legs stretched out and your arms comfortably at your sides, palms turned up. Slowly inhale and exhale through the nose, feeling your abdomen expand and contract. While you do so, start mentally scanning your body, beginning at your toes and working your way up to the top of your head, assessing whether you are holding tension anywhere. Mentally release muscular tension as you go, allowing your body, inch by inch, to comfortably sink into the surface it is lying on. You may fall asleep in the process or you might simply hold the pose for five breaths and then slowly transition into your favorite sleeping posture to fall asleep.

Don't Let Your Bed Partner Ruin Your Sleep—Simple Solutions for the Most Common Problems

Jeffry H. Larson, PhD, licensed marriage and family therapist for more than 25 years and a professor of marriage and family therapy at the College of Family, Home and Social Sciences at Brigham Young University in Provo, Utah. He is author of *Should We Stay Together? A Scientifically Proven Method for Evaluating Your Relationship and Improving Its Chances for Long-Term Success.*

Sooner or later, one in every four American couples ends up sleeping in separate beds. Maybe it's your spouse's tossing and turning or TV watching in bed. Whatever the reason, it may seem easier just to turn that spare bedroom into a nighttime sanctuary of your own. But is that arrangement healthy?

New thinking: Even with the challenges that can come with sharing a bed, the net effect is usually positive for your health. While the exact mechanism is unknown, scientists believe that sleeping with a bed partner curbs levels of the stress hormone cortisol and inflammation-promoting proteins known as cytokines...while boosting levels of the so-called "love" hormone oxytocin.

Sleeping in the same bed also cultivates feelings of intimacy and security, which can strengthen a relationship and promote better sleep—factors linked to living a longer life. *Here, six common challenges and how to overcome them...*

•**You like to keep the room dark, while your partner prefers it light.** Sleep experts recommend keeping the room dark to help stimulate the production of the naturally occurring sleep hormone melatonin.

My advice: Room-darkening shades or light-blocking curtains help create the darkness we need for a good night's rest. But if your partner insists on having some light in the room, consider placing a dim night-light near his/ her side of the bed. The person who prefers darkness may want to wear a sleep mask.

•**You're always cold, but your bed partner is too warm.** Sleep experts agree that a cooler room is generally more conducive to sleep and complements the natural temperature drop that occurs in the body when you go to sleep.

My advice: Optimal room temperature for the best sleep varies from person to person—most insomnia experts recommend a range of 60°F to 68°F. To help achieve your personal comfort level, use separate blankets so you can easily cover yourself or remove the blanket during the night without disturbing your bed partner. If you like to use an electric blanket during the winter, choose one with separate temperature controls.

•**You're a night owl, but your partner is a lark.** If the two bed partners prefer different bedtimes, this can cause both of them to lose sleep and can be a major contributor to marital strife. In a study involving 150 couples, which I conducted with several colleagues at Brigham Young University, the University of Nebraska–Lincoln and Montana State University, those who had mismatched body clocks argued more, spent less time doing shared activities and had slightly less sex.

The first step in trying to resolve conflicting bedtimes is to understand that one's circadian rhythm, the internal body clock that regulates sleep and wakefulness as well as other biological processes, dictates whether you are a natural early riser or a night owl. One's particular circadian rhythm is determined by genetics but can be influenced by sunlight, time zone changes and work schedules. Bedtime tendencies also can be socially learned.

My advice: Have a conversation with your partner. Avoid blaming the other party for having a different sleep schedule—we can't control our circadian rhythms or such factors as work schedules. Then, like everything else in a partnership, you'll need to compromise.

For instance, say your partner likes to go to bed at 10 pm and get up at 6 am, while you're rarely in bed before 1 am and sleep until 10 am. As a compromise, you might agree to get in bed with your partner at 9:30 pm to talk, snuggle, relax, read together, etc. Then, when your partner is ready to go to sleep, you can get up and continue with your night. Alternatively, you and your partner could agree to go to bed at the same time two or three nights a week. A night owl could also lie in bed and listen to music or an audiobook with headphones while his partner sleeps.

•**Your bed partner wants to watch TV, but you want peace and quiet.** Watching TV—or looking at any illuminated screen, such as a laptop or smartphone—promotes wakefulness and can interfere with sleep. So it's not really something anyone should do just before lights out. However, if one partner wants to watch TV or use a laptop before bed, he should do it in another room.

•**Your partner thrashes all night long.** Some individuals are naturally restless sleepers, tossing and turning throughout the night. Others may have restless legs syndrome (RLS) and/or periodic limb movement disorder (PLMD)—two related but distinct conditions.

RLS causes unpleasant sensations, such as tingling and burning, in the legs and an overwhelming urge to move them when the sufferer is sitting or attempting to sleep. PLMD causes involuntary movements and jerking of the limbs during sleep—the legs are most often affected but arm movements also can occur.

With RLS, the sufferer is aware of the problem. Individuals with PLMD, on the other hand, frequently are not aware that they move so much.

My advice: To help ease symptoms, you may want to try natural strategies such as taking warm baths, walking regularly and/or using magnesium supplements, which also promote sleep. But be sure to check with a doctor. If you have RLS or PLMD, it could signal an underlying health condition, such as iron deficiency.

If symptoms persist, you may want to talk to your doctor about medications such as *ropinirole* (Requip) and *pramipexole* (Mirapex), which can help relieve symptoms. Side effects may include nausea and drowsiness.

•**Your partner snores a lot—and loudly.** This is not only a nuisance, it also makes it hard for you to sleep.

My advice: In some cases, running a fan, listening to music through earbuds or using a white-noise machine can help.

If the snoring occurs almost every night, however, your partner may need to see an otolaryngologist (ear, nose and throat doctor) to determine whether there's an underlying medical condition.

Loud snoring that is accompanied by periods in which the person's breathing stops for a few seconds and then resumes may indicate sleep apnea, a serious—but treatable—disorder usually caused by a blocked or narrowed airway.

The New Anti-Snoring Workout

Murray Grossan, MD, a board-certified otolaryngologist at Tower Ear, Nose & Throat at Cedars-Sinai Medical Center in Los Angeles. He is also author of *The Whole Person Tinnitus Relief Program* (DrGrossanTinnitus.com) and founder of Hydro Med Inc.

Snoring can be a nightmare—both for the sufferer and his/her bed partner. But until recently, the treatments have been limited. A snorer might be told to lose weight, for example, wear a mouth guard or a mask (part of a continuous positive airway pressure, or CPAP, system) that delivers a steady stream of air at night…change his sleeping position…or, in severe cases, get surgery.

Recent development: In a recent study of 39 men who snored or had mild obstructive sleep apnea (OSA), a common cause of snoring, scientists found that performing mouth and tongue exercises reduced the frequency and intensity of snoring by up to 59%—a reduction on par with other therapies, including mouth guards or surgery.

And while snoring may seem like more of an annoyance than a health problem, that is simply not true. Snoring has been linked to medical conditions, including heart attack, stroke and glaucoma. *How mouth and tongue exercises can help…*

Sit-Ups for Your Throat

If your bed partner has complained of your snoring or you have unexplained daytime sleepiness, consider trying the following exercises.

About half of my patients improve enough after doing these exercises (think of them as "throat sit-ups") for five minutes three times a day for six weeks to avoid surgery or other inconvenient therapies such as wearing a mouth guard or using CPAP. They also awaken feeling more refreshed and reduce their odds of developing OSA.

Here are the main exercises included in the recent study mentioned above (led by Geraldo Lorenzi-Filho, MD, PhD)—along with some slight variations that I have found to be effective for my patients. The tongue positions for these exercises strengthen your tongue muscle and the sides of your throat. However, my variations give these muscles a more rigorous strength-training workout.

- **Tongue Push.**

What to do: Push the tip of your tongue forcefully behind your upper front teeth and move it all the way back along the roof of your mouth (palate) 20 times.

My variation: Say the vowel sounds "A, E, I, O, U" while doing the exercise.

- **Flat Tongue Press.**

What to do: Suck your tongue up against the roof of your mouth, pressing the entire tongue against your palate 20 times.

My variation: Repeat "A, E, I, O, U" while doing the exercise.

- **Say "Ahhh."**

What to do: Focus on raising the back of the roof of the mouth and uvula (the fleshy appendage in the throat that's responsible for the rattling sound made by snorers) 20 times.

My variation: Say the vowel "A" (or "Ahhh") while doing the exercise.

These Therapies Help, Too

Colds, allergies and sinus infections can cause nasal congestion and/or postnasal drip—two common conditions that can make your throat swell, increasing your risk for snoring. *What helps…*

- **Nasal lavage (using a saline solution to irrigate and cleanse the nasal cavity) helps clear nasal congestion and postnasal drip.** Subjects in the study mentioned above performed nasal lavage three times a day. Based on my clinical experience, once a day does the job.

A product that I created called The Hydro Pulse Sinus System ($99.99, HydroMedOnline.com) works well. It includes a special throat attachment that directs pulsating irrigation to the tonsils and throat to ease swelling. But you could also use a neti pot (typical cost: $14.99)—just be sure to keep it clean and sanitized between uses and use distilled or sterile water to prevent a sinus infection. Or you can buy sterile squeeze bottles filled with nasal saline.

•**Nose taping.** With age, the tip of one's nose naturally begins to droop some. This can obstruct the nasal valve, which impedes breathing and contributes to snoring.

Try this simple test: Use your finger to press the tip of your nose up. If breathing feels easier when you do this, try taping your nose up before bedtime.

What to do: Cut a three-inch strip of one-half-inch medical grade tape. Place it under the nose at the center, without blocking the airway. Gently lift the nose as you run the tape up the midline of the nose to the area between the eyes. The taping should be comfortable and is for use during sleep.

Important: Commercial nasal strips, such as Breathe Right, spread the sides of the nose apart. Taping up the nose, as described above, also does this, with the additional advantage of opening the nasal valve.

Hidden Brain Dangers of Sleep Apnea... Especially for Women

Paul M. Macey, PhD, assistant professor in residence, associate dean for information technology and innovation, School of Nursing, University of California, Los Angeles. His study was published in *PLoS ONE.*

You probably know that obstructive sleep apnea causes people to gasp, snort and snore as their sleep is interrupted by repeated stops and starts in their breathing. And you know that these mini-suffocations, which can occur dozens of times each hour, increase the risk for all kinds of serious health problems.

But you probably don't know that sleep apnea causes permanent changes to the structure of the brain and how the brain controls blood pressure. These changes create a vicious cycle that leaves apnea patients starved for oxygen not only at night, but also during the day—particularly at times when their bodies are most in need of oxygen!

Though sleep apnea often is thought of as a "man's problem," women develop it, too...and women are at especially high risk for the dangerous nervous system changes, a recent study reveals. Male or female, if you (or a loved one) have or may have sleep apnea, you need to know about this research...

Autonomic Glitch

Participants in the recent study included male and female patients who recently had been diagnosed with sleep apnea and were not receiving treatment, plus some healthy "controls" (people without sleep apnea who served as a basis of comparison).

The point of the experiment was to see how people's bodies respond to various physical "challenges" that use different nervous system pathways to signal increased cardiovascular demand. These challenges mimic day-to-day activities, such as straining, lifting and touching something cold. Normally such challenges, like many everyday activities, cause heart rate to speed up. This is a protective response of the autonomic regulatory system (the part of the central nervous system that regulates heart rate, blood pressure, breathing, etc. without you having to think about it), sending extra blood and oxygen to cells that are in greater need.

The challenges in the experiment included a hand-grip task (squeezing an inflatable bag with one hand as hard as possible for 16 seconds)…keeping a foot in icy water for one minute…and breathing out hard with the mouth closed and nose pinched shut (similar to what happens when a person is straining over a bowel movement).

Results: For all three challenges, compared with the healthy controls, the sleep apnea patients showed an impaired response—meaning that they had heart rate increases that were less pronounced and slower to kick in.

Also, in comparing male sleep apnea patients with female sleep apnea patients, the researchers found that the degree of impairment was worse in women. Take the bag-squeezing test, for example. The heart rate of women with apnea increased just 3.3% and returned to normal very quickly, whereas in healthy women, heart rate increased 5.8% and remained elevated significantly longer. For men, however, the differences between those with and without apnea were much less pronounced. Heart rate increased 7.4% in apnea patients, compared with 8.6% in healthy men…and there was only a small difference in how long it remained elevated in the two male groups.

Why such an impaired response is dangerous: An impaired response means that tissues, including sensitive brain cells, are being starved of oxygen because blood flow is inadequate. Obviously, sleep apnea patients are oxygen-deprived whenever they stop breathing during sleep—but this study shows that people with sleep apnea also often are deprived of oxygen when they are awake and during daily physical tasks, when oxygen is needed most.

That's because their nervous systems don't do a good job of increasing heart rate as needed to meet demands at times when the body is physiologically challenged.

What's more, this impaired response creates a vicious cycle—impaired blood flow leads to structural changes in the brain and cardiovascular system, which leads to further impaired blood flow—and so on. The worse this gets, the greater the risk may be for heart disease, high blood pressure and other chronic illnesses associated with autonomic dysfunction, the study researchers noted. While both male and female sleep apnea patients are at risk, the dangers for women may be particularly high, given their greater magnitude of autonomic response impairment and the fact that they are less likely to be properly diagnosed in the first place.

Self-defense for women and men: Sleep apnea affects an estimated 28 million adults in the US, more than 80% of whom do not realize that they have the disorder. If you have been told that you snore, gasp or grunt as you sleep, or if you often feel groggy during the day even after a full night's rest, ask your doctor about being tested for sleep apnea. Early detection and treatment can help protect against damage to the brain, cardiovascular system and other organs...and allow you to sleep better and feel better, too.

How to Finally Fix Your Sleep Apnea

Michael Breus, PhD, a sleep specialist in private practice in Scottsdale, Arizona, and author of *Good Night: The Sleep Doctor's 4-Week Program to Better Sleep and Better Health.* He is a Diplomate of the American Board of Sleep Medicine and a Fellow of the American Academy of Sleep Medicine.

If you've got obstructive sleep apnea (OSA)—that well-known sleep disorder marked by snoring and gasping—you've no doubt been told that it's a serious condition. It can lead to high blood pressure, heart disease and stroke, along with severe fatigue and night after night of disrupted sleep.

In case that all sounds pretty frightening, don't lose hope. OSA can be virtually eliminated with a nondrug treatment. The problem is, about half of all patients stop using the treatment within the first year. Some last only a few nights.

Why do so many people give up on a treatment that works so well? Because they hate it!

However, there are ways to make "CPAP"—the nickname of this treatment—much more tolerable so that you can finally get the pleasant sleep you need and deserve.

Here's how to make CPAP a much better experience...

Treatment That Works

The gold standard treatment for sleep apnea is continuous positive airway pressure (CPAP). With this therapy, a machine about the size of a shoe box delivers a constant flow of air that opens your airways and improves your breathing.

Unfortunately, CPAP machine users are tethered to the machine all night, and some of these machines are noisy. You also have to wear a mask over your mouth and/or nose, which makes some people claustrophobic. And the flow of air can cause uncomfortable mouth/nose dryness and eye irritation.

Startling study: Only 46% of patients prescribed CPAP used the devices for more than four hours a night on 70% of all nights—the threshold for effective treatment.

Because proper use of CPAP can reduce health risks associated with sleep apnea to close to zero, this is not a treatment that you want to give up if you have this condition.

Making Peace With CPAP

If you're prescribed CPAP therapy, you may want to start out with a basic machine just to see how well you respond. Ask your respiratory therapist about renting a machine to try it out first. This device might do a good job of improving your symptoms, and the purchase price is usually $500 or less, compared with pricier, more sophisticated units (see below).

But what if you find the machine to be so uncomfortable that you stop using it? You have a lot of options. A sleep specialist or respiratory therapist can help you sort them out. CPAP machines are usually covered by insurance. *Where to start...*

•**Different masks.** A full-face style that covers the mouth and nose provides a good fit and is more likely than other masks to stay put during the night. A total face mask extends all the way from the forehead to the chin. But you'll look like Darth Vader and might, ironically, feel like you're suffocating.

You may prefer a nasal "pillow," an under-the-nose mask with nostril tubes that's less obtrusive and won't obscure your vision if you like to read before falling asleep.

A nasal mask that fits only over the nose is yet another choice. It's more likely than the nasal pillow to stay in place. Many people find this more comfortable than a full-face configuration. Prices for the masks described above generally range from $40 to $200 (in addition to the cost of a CPAP machine).

•**A "ramp" feature.** Most CPAP machines, starting at around $500, have a feature that gradually ramps up air pressure so that the full force won't be felt right away. The machine can be programmed to automatically raise pressure every five minutes or so until the prescribed amount is reached—and you have fallen asleep.

•**Heated humidification.** This is now a standard feature on many units. Everyone who uses CPAP occasionally suffers from nose or mouth dryness. The humidity added by certain machines reduces this effect and makes you more comfortable. You need to fill and clean a water tank with these models. They are available at all price levels, from less than $500 to more than $1,500.

Also helpful: A squirt of saline solution into each nostril before you put on any CPAP mask. Doing this will help prevent dryness and nighttime congestion.

•**Bilevel PAP.** Unlike the continuous pressure in some machines, bilevel PAP (also known as BiPAP) units match the airflow to your breathing. They increase pressure during inhalations—when apneas (breathing cessations) usually occur—and decrease it when you exhale. Research has shown that people with bilevel PAP machines are more likely to keep using them than those with non-bilevel PAP units. Prices start at about $600.

•**AutoPAP.** These machines are a bit different from bilevel PAP machines because they automatically change air pressure on a breath-by-breath basis. When you sleep on your back, for example, you will naturally tend to have more apneas. The machine will detect breathing changes and make the necessary adjustments in air pressure. Prices start at around $400.

"No More CPAP!"

Some people never get comfortable using CPAP of any kind. For these individuals—especially if they have milder OSA—other options include...

•**Oral appliance.** This custom-made mouthpiece helps keep the airway open and is especially effective for people who sleep on their backs. The $1,800 to $2,000 cost may be covered by insurance.

•**Nasal valves.** When you go to bed, you apply a small, Band-Aid–like strip over each nasal opening. The strips have nasal plugs with small valves. The valves open when you inhale, then partially close when you breathe out. This creates expiratory positive airway pressure that helps keep the airways open.

Example: Provent Sleep Apnea Therapy. This FDA-approved sleep apnea treatment requires a prescription and costs about $60 a month, which might not be covered by insurance. It may not be suitable for people with chronic health conditions such as heart disease.

CPAP Alternative

Karl Franklin, MD, senior lecturer, Umea University, Sweden.

A customized oral appliance that moves the jawbone slightly forward during sleep helps keep the airway open and may work better for some adults who cannot tolerate a continuous positive airway pressure (CPAP) mask and machine.

Recent finding: Nearly 100 adults with mild-to-moderate sleep apnea who wore this type of mouth guard nightly showed improvement in sleep apnea and snoring.

If you've been diagnosed with sleep apnea: Ask your doctor whether an oral appliance would be appropriate. If so, a dentist can custom-fit one. Most devices cost about $2,000 and may be covered by insurance.

CHAPTER 10

How Your Brain Can Heal Your Body

The Mind-Body Cure for Chronic Pain Helps Headaches, Back Pain and More

John E. Sarno, MD, who died in 2017, was professor of clinical rehabilitation medicine at New York University School of Medicine and an attending physician at The Rusk Institute of Rehabilitation Medicine, both in New York City. He wrote several best-selling books, including *Healing Back Pain: The Mind-Body Connection* and *The Divided Mind: The Epidemic of Mindbody Disorders.*

From backaches and headaches to wrist pain caused by carpal tunnel syndrome, chronic pain continues to be an enormous problem in this country. Why is that? Because the average doctor persists in the mistaken belief that pain is a structural disorder.

It's now quite clear that most chronic pain is the result of an emotionally induced physical condition—which, in turn, is the result of hidden conflict between our conscious and unconscious minds.

This mind-body cycle of pain is known as tension myositis syndrome (TMS).

Three-Step Sequence

Chronic pain typically occurs as a result of a three-step sequence…

1. You're under pressure. It might be psychological stress caused by perfectionism or another self-induced pressure…or an external pressure, such as a demanding boss.

2. Growing pressure gives rise to rage and frustration. These feelings lie within the unconscious mind only. That's because they're simply too frightening to be acceptable to your conscious mind. You're not even aware of their existence—despite the fact that they can be very intense.

3. To keep angry feelings from spilling over into consciousness, your subconscious mind directs your attention to your body. It does so by activating your autonomic nervous system, which controls digestion, respiration, circulation and other involuntary functions. Upon activation, the autonomic nervous system reduces blood flow to a particular muscle, tendon of nerve. Exactly which part of the body is affected varies. The decrease in circulation deprives the tissues of oxygen. That causes pain.

Stopping Chronic Pain

To stop pain caused by TMS, you don't need painkilling medication...or surgery...or physical therapy. What you need is an understanding of the three-step sequence. Once you acknowledge that pain stems from the subconscious mind's efforts to protect your conscious mind from troubling emotions, you can get on with the cure...

•**Have a doctor rule out physical causes.** You must be absolutely certain that there is no serious disease causing your pain—cancer, for example.

Important: Despite what many doctors believe, spinal disc abnormalities are rarely the cause of back pain. In a 1984 study, back-pain sufferers proved to be no more likely to have spinal disc degeneration or bone spurs than people who did not have back pain. In a similar study, researchers detected disc abnormalities in 64 people—none of whom had back pain.

•**"Talk" to your brain.** This sounds silly, but it works. If you feel a twinge of pain, silently tell your brain that you know what it is doing—you can even tell it to increase the blood flow to the painful area. Put your brain on notice that you're no longer going to let yourself be affected by its efforts to shield you from negative emotions.

Accept that pain is caused by repressed emotions. It can be very hard to admit that emotions are causing your pain—especially if a doctor has told you that the culprit is a slipped disc or another structural problem...or physical stress, such as that caused by typing for hours a day. Of course, your conscious mind is desperately trying to deny that emotions are the cause. It doesn't want to experience those emotions—or even admit they exist.

•**Make a written list of the possible sources of your psychological stress.** In making the list, remember that most distress is internally generated. *Two common examples...*

Example #1: Perfectionism. Because you're so eager to excel at everything you do, you're highly critical of yourself—and overly sensitive to criticism from others.

Example #2: The need to be liked. You try to be good and nice to everyone—because you want everyone's love, admiration and respect. "Goodism" is just as stressful as perfectionism—and just as likely to cause frustration and rage.

External causes of distress might include a mean boss, an argumentative spouse, a meddlesome relative or another person with whom you have a difficult relationship.

It could also be serious financial trouble or simply a sense of having too little time to get things done.

Even happy experiences—marriage, job promotion, a new baby—create pressure. And pressure creates unconscious rage.

By reading and rereading your list—and reminding yourself of the true cause of your pain—you'll "cure" the pain. Most people who use this technique become pain-free within eight weeks.

•**Review your list on a daily basis.** Spend at least 30 minutes a day thinking about each item on your list and how it could be causing pressure in your life. Resolve to take action to defuse the pressures you can change...and to accept the pressures you cannot change.

•**Visualize your rage.** Imagine yourself in a blind fury. That is the experience your unconscious mind is having to cope with on a continuing basis. Now consider what might happen if you gave free rein to your rage. You could ruin your marriage, lose your job—even wind up in jail. Your conscious mind is as frightened of these experiences as you are. That's why it chooses to hide your rage from you.

•**Resume physical activity.** Once your pain has largely subsided, go back to exercising, lifting heavy objects, using a computer keyboard, etc. Start slowly, and build up over a period of weeks.

If you're afraid to resume normal activity, it means that your unconscious mind is still in charge. You've got more mind-body work to do.

•**Understand "location substitution."** Say you've just gotten over a bad case of back pain—and now your elbow has started to hurt. Chances are that the brain has simply picked a new spot in your body to cause pain to distract you from your rage. Realize the same pain process is happening once again—only in another part of your body. Once again, the pain should disappear.

Stay Pain-Free Forever

To keep pain at bay, you must continually remind yourself that pressure causes unconscious, frightening rage…and your brain distracts your attention from that rage by creating pain. Tell yourself this again and again, and you should stay pain-free for the rest of your life.

Grow a Happy Brain

Richard O'Connor, PhD, psychotherapist in private practice, Canaan, Connecticut, and New York City. He is former executive director of the Northwest Center for Family Service and Mental Health and author of *Undoing Depression: What Therapy Doesn't Teach You and Medication Can't Give You.* UndoingDepression.com

About three-quarters of patients who are treated for depression take one or more antidepressant medications. In fact, about 10% of all Americans are taking these drugs.

Antidepressants, including Prozac and other selective serotonin reuptake inhibitors (SSRIs), can help patients with severe depression, but they are not effective for most patients with mild-to-moderate depression. A recent report in *The Journal of the American Medical Association* concluded that some of the most widely prescribed antidepressants are no more effective than placebos for these patients.

Also, these drugs commonly cause sexual problems, weight gain and other side effects, including an inability to feel empathy for others. These side effects might be acceptable for someone who is incapacitated with depression, but the risk-benefit ratio isn't acceptable for the types of depression that can be treated with other methods. Here's how to relieve depression without taking medications.

Important: Never stop taking an antidepressant without your doctor's approval, and be sure to taper off slowly.

Grow a Happy Brain

It has been discovered in recent years that chronic depression causes significant brain damage. Patients produce less dopamine, one of the neurotransmitters that affects the ability to feel pleasure. The hippocampus, one part of the brain associated with emotions, can shrink by up to 20%. Cells lose endorphin (the pleasure hormone) receptor sites, which further inhibits pleasurable feelings.

Good news: Much of this damage can be reversed with positive emotions—by trying the strategies in this article and continuing to use the ones that work for you. Just as the areas of the brain associated with hand coordination get larger when a musician practices his/her instrument, people with depression can increase the areas of the brain associated with positive emotions.

Keep Track

Sudden mood changes can be a hallmark of depression. The dramatic ups and downs that some patients experience are triggered by unfelt feelings. Because of their past experiences (such as childhood trauma), they have learned to mute their feelings—experiencing them is too painful.

Example: You might go to bed feeling fine, then wake up in the throes of depression. You are reacting to something, but because you don't know what that something is, you feel buffeted by forces beyond your control.

Solution: A mood journal. Every day, keep track of what's happening when you experience any type of mood change. Write down what you're feeling, what you were doing when you first noticed the feeling and what you were thinking about or remembering at the time.

This is a powerful tool to help you circumvent your defense mechanisms. You will start to recognize more of your feelings and understand why you're having them. This won't make the emotional pain disappear (you might even feel more upset when you first start doing this), but you will start to recognize emotional causes and effects. This knowledge will lead to solutions as well as a greater sense of control.

Do Something

Patients with severe depression can be almost catatonic—just getting out of bed or taking a shower can seem impossible. With milder forms of depression, procrastination is one of the biggest hurdles. Starting something is risky. There might be failure. There will be frustrations and setbacks. Self-esteem may be threatened. Doing nothing can feel like a safer alternative even though the lack of accomplishment will make the depression worse.

People don't accomplish things because they are naturally productive and energetic. They become productive and energetic by doing things.

Solution: Every day, make yourself do something that gives you a sense of accomplishment. You might make a commitment to work in the yard or fix a garden fence. You might decide to write a few lines of a poem.

It doesn't matter what the activity is, as long as you do something. People who set goals and deadlines (I'm going to write for 10 minutes tomorrow at 10 am) and follow through almost always notice an improvement in mood. Once they experience that uplift, they are more likely to keep trying new things.

Get Off the Roller Coaster

Depression is accompanied by thought patterns that are rife with distorted perceptions and faulty logic.

Example: A healthy individual who gets a flat tire will focus on the immediate problem—*Darn, I have a flat tire. I'll have to get it fixed.*

Someone with depression will imagine the worst possible scenario. *All of my tires must be going bad. I don't have the money to replace them all. I might have to get another job...*

They get so worked up that they forget they are dealing with a simple problem. Instead, the imaginary scenario dominates their thinking.

Solution: Take yourself off the mental roller coaster. When you start imagining the worst, think *Stop.* Ask yourself how likely any of these dire outcomes really is. Once people understand that they're prone to making exaggerated—and erroneous—generalizations, they find it easier to mentally step back and focus on the real problem. *Oh, it's just a flat tire. It feels like a huge problem, but it's not.*

Watch Your Mind

Studies have found that people who practice mindful meditation—noting the thoughts that run through their minds without letting those thoughts upset them—have increased activity in the prefrontal part of the brain. This is where positive emotions are processed and negative emotions are controlled.

Mindfulness means watching your mind at work. You are aware of yourself and your thoughts, but you are detached from the emotional components. People who practice mindfulness become more thoughtful about their emotions and are less likely to react to them.

This is critical for people with depression. They tend to ruminate too much. They worry about things that haven't happened and attach too much importance to things that don't matter.

Solution: Daily meditation. Find a quiet place where you won't be interrupted for 20 or 30 minutes. Get comfortable, close your eyes and start to breathe slowly and deeply. Focus only on your breathing. As thoughts or feelings drift in and out of your mind, acknowledge them, then let them float off, like bubbles in a pool of water. Whenever you get distracted, return your mind to your breathing.

Don't expect to experience bliss—that's not the purpose. It's more like exercise for the brain. People who do this daily find that they're generally calmer and more resilient against stress. They learn to detach from their emotions long enough to think about what those feelings really mean and how important (or unimportant) they are.

Walk It Off

Studies of depressed adults show that those who exercise three times a week improve just as much in the short-term as those who take antidepressants. People who continue to exercise are more likely to avoid future depressive episodes than those who rely solely on medication.

Exercise appears to stimulate the growth of new brain cells, the opposite of what happens with depression. It stimulates the production of endorphins. It also promotes feelings of accomplishment and physical well-being.

Solution: Walk briskly three or more times a week. You will probably notice significant improvement in mood within the first week. Those who exercise harder or more often tend to report the greatest improvement.

How to Quiet Your Mind to Heal Disease

Norman E. Rosenthal, MD, clinical professor of psychiatry at Georgetown University School of Medicine, who maintains a private practice in the Washington, DC, area. He has conducted research at the National Institutes of Mental Health and is a recipient of the Anna-Monika Foundation Prize for his contribution to research in treating depression. He is author of *Transcendence: Healing and Transformation Through Transcendental Meditation.* NormanRosenthal.com

Wouldn't it be great if there were a simple way to lower blood pressure, reverse heart disease and sharpen your brain? There is! It's called transcendental meditation, or TM for short.

Many people think of TM as a vestige of the 1960s, a vaguely religious practice that was popularized when the Beatles went to India to study with Maharishi Mahesh Yogi.

TM is not a religious practice. It does not involve immersing yourself in a particular belief system. It's a mental technique that changes brain wave patterns and alters, in beneficial ways, physiological processes, such as blood pressure, heart rate and hormone levels.

Bonus: TM is easier to do than many other forms of meditation and relaxation therapy. And beginners exhibit the same brain wave changes as long-time practitioners, sometimes within just a few weeks after starting TM.

What It Involves

Various relaxation techniques require you to sit with your eyes closed, focus on your breathing and/or visualize a particular scene. TM requires the repetition of a mantra, a meaningless word that you mentally focus on.

There's nothing mystical about the mantra. It's simply a tool for quieting the mind and "transcending" stressful thoughts, worries and concerns.

Most people who practice TM do so twice a day for 20 minutes each time. During a session, the breathing slows and the brain (as measured on an EEG) produces a preponderance of alpha waves, slow frequency signals (eight to 12 cycles per second) that indicate deep relaxation. There's also an increase in brain wave coherence, in which activity in different parts of the brain is roughly synchronized.

TM has been studied more than most other forms of meditation and relaxation—and, in some cases, appears to have more pronounced health effects. Researchers have published approximately 340 peer-reviewed articles on TM, many of which appeared in respected medical journals. Important benefits...

Lowers Blood Pressure

A University of Kentucky meta-analysis that looked at data from 711 participants found that those who practiced TM averaged a five-point reduction in systolic pressure (top number) and three points in diastolic (bottom number). This might sound like a modest benefit, but it's enough to potentially reduce the incidence of cardiovascular disease by 15% to 20%.

Scientists speculate that TM lowers blood pressure by reducing the body's output of hormones, such as epinephrine, that accompany and stimulate the natural stress response. People with hypertension who meditate twice a day for more than three months require, on average, 23% less blood pressure medication.

Other nondrug treatments for hypertension, including biofeedback, progressive relaxation and stress-management training, don't have these same effects.

Reverses Heart Disease

Researchers divided participants with hypertension into two groups. Those in one group were given health education (the control group), while those in the second group practiced TM for six to nine months. The thickness of the intima (inner lining) of the carotid artery was measured at the beginning and end of the study.

Result: The intima thickened slightly in the control group, indicating that cardiovascular disease had progressed. In the TM group, the thickness of the intima decreased. This study, published in Stroke, indicates that TM actually can reverse cardiovascular disease.

It's not known why TM has this effect. We suspect that it's more effective in patients with early-stage disease. In those with advanced atherosclerosis, which is accompanied by calcification of plaques (fatty deposits) in the coronary arteries, TM might slow disease progression but is unlikely to remove plaque that has already accumulated.

Reduces Pain

I sometimes recommend TM for patients who suffer from chronic-pain conditions, such as arthritis. We know that pain tends to be more severe in patients with high levels of anxiety and stress—and TM is very effective at reducing stress.

In one study, participants dipped their fingers into painfully hot water, then rated the pain. Those who practiced TM rated their pain exactly the same as those who didn't use TM, but they were less bothered by it. Interestingly, participants who practiced TM for just five months achieved the same results as those who had meditated for decades.

Sharpens Your Brain

When people meditate, the coherence of alpha brain waves throughout the brain is accompanied by slightly faster beta waves in the prefrontal region of the brain, behind the forehead. The alpha waves produce relaxation, while the beta waves increase focus and decision-making.

Brain studies of top-level managers show that they have higher levels of both alpha and beta coherence than lower-level workers. A similar thing occurs in elite athletes.

Practice helps: Some of the physiological changes produced by TM occur immediately, but people who keep doing it for several months tend to have better results, probably because of increased synaptic connections (connections between brain cells). The brain may literally rewire itself, with practice.

How to Start

During a TM session, you'll achieve a state of restful alertness, during which your thoughts are clear but without the distractions of the internal noise that we live with. How people achieve this is highly individual. I like to relax in a comfortable chair in a quiet room. I dim the lights, turn off the telephones and start repeating my mantra. A friend of mine who has practiced TM for 40 years can enjoy a brief session in the back of a taxi.

You might find it tricky to keep mentally repeating the mantra. You might be distracted by physical sensations, outside sounds, etc. All of this is natural and expected. At some point during the session, you'll feel mentally silent. You will be present in the moment but removed from it.

Important: TM is easy to practice but difficult to learn on your own. People start with one-on-one sessions with an instructor. In general, each teaching session lasts about 90 minutes. Your instructor will assign a mantra and give instructions for using it. Sometimes people wonder why they can't pick their own mantras. One reason is that it is a tradition not to. Another is that someone who chooses his/her own mantra might do so because of underlying meanings or associations. A mantra from a teacher won't have this baggage.

You will work with the instructor once a day for four consecutive days. After that, you might return once every month to make sure that your technique is working. The website TM.org can provide referrals to instructors in your area.

How Meditation Can Help Arthritis, Asthma and Other Inflammation Problems

Melissa A. Rosenkranz, PhD, associate scientist, Waisman Laboratory for Brain Imaging and Behavior and Center for Investigating Healthy Minds, University of Wisconsin, Madison. Her study was published in *Brain, Behavior, and Immunity.*

Stress is bad for everybody—but particularly for people who suffer from a chronic inflammatory condition such as asthma, rheumatoid arthritis or inflammatory bowel disease. That's because stress contributes to inflammation...so it makes sense to take steps to reduce stress.

A particular type of stress-reducing technique appears to be uniquely beneficial when it comes to quelling inflammation, according to recent research. Best of all, this technique requires no drugs (or any foreign substance, for that matter)...it's easy to do...and it can be done anywhere.

How the study was done: Healthy volunteers were divided into two groups. One group was instructed in mindfulness-based stress reduction (MBSR), a technique in which a person meditates by focusing attention on his breathing and bodily sensations while sitting still, walking or doing yoga. The thing to notice is that this sort of meditation emphasizes mindfulness—which means to foster an awareness of each sensation, emotion or thought as it unfolds in the moment, catching and then releasing it without judgment. The other group participated in a program that combined physical activity, music therapy and instruction in improved nutrition—all of which are known to improve well-being but do not include the idea of mindfulness. Both groups received the same amount of training and did the same amount of at-home practice for eight weeks.

Before starting and again after the end of the eight-week programs, the researchers provoked stress in the participants by asking them to give short impromptu speeches and to do some mental arithmetic problems. Next, a cream with an irritant was placed on the participants' forearms to induce inflammation, then a sucking device was applied to raise blisters. This allowed the researchers to collect some fluid from the irritated skin so that levels of two cytokines (proteins released by the immune system) could be measured. Researchers also measured the size of the resulting inflamed areas of skin and the amount of the stress hormone cortisol secreted in the participants' saliva at various times throughout the day.

Results: It was not surprising that the stress caused by giving speeches and doing mental math caused increases in markers for stress—and the levels of the cytokines and cortisol were about the same in both groups. But: Participants who had practiced mindfulness meditation showed significantly less stress-induced inflammation (as measured by the area of inflamed skin) than those in the other group…and their cortisol levels on a normal day showed a healthier circadian rhythm.

In other words, the meditators had reduced their bodies' inflammatory response—something that would be good for anyone, but that could provide an especially profound health benefit for a person with an inflammatory condition!

Bottom line: If you have a chronic inflammatory health problem—or if you want an extra measure of protection against the harmful effects of inflammation—consider taking a class in mindfulness meditation. It's a very popular sort of meditation, and you shouldn't have trouble finding a class in your area. Or visit the website of the University of Massachusetts Center for Mindfulness in Medicine, Health Care, and Society to search for an MBSR-trained practitioner near you.

The Healing Power of Compassion

Charles Raison, MD, clinical director, Mind-Body Program, Emory University School of Medicine…and former Tibetan Buddhist monk Geshe Lobsang Tenzin Negi, PhD, senior lecturer, Emory University, and spiritual director, Drepung Loseling Monastery, all in Atlanta.

Thinking empathetically about other people improves your own health, research shows. Regularly meditating on the well-being of others reduces your body's inflammatory responses to stress—and that lowers your risk for heart disease, diabetes, dementia and other stress-related health problems.

The goal of compassion meditation is to reshape your responses to other people by concentrating on the interconnectedness of every human being.

It's easy: Try the following technique for 10 minutes a day, three to four times per week.

•**Week One.** Sit comfortably, eyes closed, breathing deeply. Think about a time when you were kind to another person—for instance, helping a loved one through a crisis or simply holding a door for a stranger. Recognize your great capacity for goodness. For the last few minutes of your meditation, repeat, "May I be free from suffering…may I find the sources of happiness."

•**Week Two.** Repeat the same exercise, this time building compassion toward a loved one. Think about someone close to you—your mother, daughter, dear friend—and focus on what a blessing she is in your life. Then think about any suffering she is experiencing...and what you can do to ease her pain.

Recite: "May she be free from suffering...may she find the sources of happiness."

•**Week Three.** Think about someone with whom you have only a minor connection—a bus driver, a waiter at your favorite café. How is he a blessing in your life? How might he be suffering? How can you ease his pain (for instance, with a smile and a sincere word of thanks)? Conclude with the recitation.

•**Week Four.** Focus on someone you dislike—a whiny neighbor, a critical cousin. Identify blessings, perhaps as lessons you have learned about being patient or not judging others. Consider how the person may suffer...for instance, from being a quitter or having few friends. Finish with the recitation.

•**Moving Ahead.** Continue to practice several times weekly, incorporating all four types of compassion into your meditation.

Index